W9-BIS-175

MOVE THE BODY, HEAL THE MIND

MOVE THE BODY, HEAL THE MIND

Overcome Anxiety, Depression, and
Dementia and Improve Focus,
Creativity, and Sleep

Jennifer J. Heisz, PhD

MARINER BOOKS

Boston   New York

Photography © 2022 by Paulina Rzeczkowska

marinerbooks.com

Library of Congress Cataloging-in-Publication Data has been applied for.
ISBN 978-0-358-57340-1 (hbk)
ISBN 978-0-358-57383-8 (ebk)

Book design by Laura Shaw Design

Printed in the United States of America
1 2022
4500846787

To my darling daughter Monica,
may you never live in fear or suffer alone.

AUTHOR'S NOTE

Thank you for joining me on this journey toward better health. In this book you'll find a collection of my original research and favorite studies that reveal how to move the body to heal the mind. The information provided in this book is based on research and is for educational and informational purposes only. It is made available to you as a self-help tool and is not intended to replace advice from your health care provider. Although exercise has tremendous benefits, there is a possibility of physical injury, and in participating in these workouts, you do so at your own risk. Because of this, I highly recommend that you consult with your physician prior to starting any new exercise program.

This book includes case study characters who are an amalgam of the average person in the study. I've also included case studies of famous people who have courageously shared their personal stories in the public domain. Although I would love to meet these people someday, the stories included in this book are based on secondary sources from interviews and media quotes.

The stories about me are true with the exception of my interactions with the fictional characters from the studies. Stories about my family and friends are real. However, in some cases their names have been changed.

I hope this book will teach you how to better care for your body and mind and inspire you to move a little more.

Yours in good health,
Dr. Heisz

CONTENTS

INTRODUCTION

The Healing Power of Exercise

Every new beginning comes from some other beginning's end.

— SENECA

HERE WE GO, on the cusp of a new journey! Time to move the body and heal the mind — soothe your anxiety, ease your pain, fix your depression, keep you sober, prevent dementia, alleviate your insomnia, find your focus, and optimize your creativity. Sounds great. I'm in!

But wait . . . something's wrong.

You're not quite ready.

Stuck. Full stop. Hesitant to begin again.

Don't worry.

You are not alone.

The first few steps on any new fitness journey are the most difficult.

But I promise it does get easier.

How do I know?

I've been my own guinea pig on a journey from sedentary scholar to triathlete. Along the way I've discovered the unexpected benefits of exercise on my own brain that are upheld by ground-breaking science. I'm excited to share with you all that I have discovered in the hopes that it will help you on your own journey, whether it is to start exercising, enhance your current fitness level, or go for gold.

But this book is not just about exercise and the brain. It's about navigating life. My life has been full of moments where it's been hard to breathe. I breathe easier now, and I want that for you. Exercise was my antidote. **I needed to move my body to heal my mind.**

In this **self-help guide on the neuroscience of exercise**, I share with you exactly how it worked for me. My evidence-based how-to approach will help you enhance your own brain health through exercise. You will emerge fully equipped with an exercise skill set to help you achieve greater resiliency, a more positive outlook, sharper focus, enhanced productivity, and more meaningful relationships. Yes, you can have it all!

But before we embark on this journey together, I must warn you.

To harness the healing power of exercise . . . you actually have to do it.

I know, easier said than done.

So, let's *ease* into things together.

Let's begin where it all began for me, 3 years, 8 months, and 24 days ago. It was the beginning of an end. And as you will see, it was awfully difficult for me to get started.

MY BEGINNING'S END

It was New Year's Eve, December 31, 2016. The party was at our house, but I was in no condition to host. I had a secret, and its burden was becoming too heavy for me to carry alone.

My marriage was ~~ending~~ over. But how could I admit that to anyone? They were all there when I said, "Until death do us part." And at the time, I had wholly meant it. But things had changed, promises were broken, and there was no love left.

At the stroke of midnight, we exchanged a dry peck. I had officially lost my liveliness in the loneliness of this marriage. I used to be a deeply passionate person. Long romantic kisses were my favorite. On that night, with that kiss, I was so far removed from who I was that I worried that if I didn't break free soon, my true self would be gone forever.

It would still take me months to leave him. The stress of the situation had weakened my body to the point of frailty. I doubted whether I could make it on my own. I needed time to restore my strength. To break down the illusion of dependency so I could finally be free from the suffocating situation.

For the time being, I wore a fake smile to veil my secret and prayed for the promise of something new, something real, something I could get excited about.

A love affair? That would surely jolt me back to life, but I was still married.

Cut my hair? Nah, I tried that before, and it didn't make me feel any better.

And then, it came to me in the form of a New Year's resolution. A tradition I had upheld every year. I usually resolved to be more productive at work or more helpful at home, but that year I decided to choose something just for myself.

The resolution?

A new fitness goal (I know, zero points for originality).

But not just any fitness goal: a triathlon.

Could I do it? Probably. But if you had asked me 10 years earlier, the answer would have been a definite no. The truth is I have never been an athlete. I was overweight in elementary school. I could still hear the ridicule of my classmates: "It ain't over till the fat lady sings. Come on, Jen, sing!" When I hit puberty, I became obsessed with thinness and developed a serious eating disorder that nearly destroyed my body. My late teens and early twenties were marked with several failed attempts at becoming a runner. Then, on a whim, I borrowed a friend's rusty old road bike and fell in love with cycling. At the time, it was just a nice escape from my studies. I didn't realize it then, but those bike rides started me on a new path where I would gain the physical fitness I needed to transform from sedentary scholar to triathlete and the mental toughness I needed to survive the next decade of my life. My newfound exercise had strengthened my body and my mind.

That rusty old road bike also inspired a shift in my professional life. At the time, I was completing my doctorate in neuroscience, researching how tiny brain cells use electrical impulses to represent "who we are." As I pedaled my way through my PhD and into my postdoctoral training, the movement sparked a shift in my research toward exercise. In 2013, I joined the department of kinesiology at McMaster University and founded the NeuroFit Lab, where I began intense study on the impact of exercise on the brain. Throughout this book I present our latest research, highlighting the incredible interplay between the mind and the body that can be harnessed by exercise to transform your life.

And on that eve of 2017, I needed a transformation more than ever. So, with a glass of Champagne in my hand and hope in my heart, I made a toast to the first chapter of my new life.

1

THE REASONS IT'S HARD TO EXERCISE

Start where you are. Use what you have. Do what you can.

— ARTHUR ASHE

NEW YEAR! NEW YOU! Your motivation is high and your effort is strong.

In the beginning, exercising is easy.

But then . . . it's not.

Three times a week becomes two and then one.

Suddenly, you're too busy to exercise and too tired to move; at least, that's what the brain wants you to believe. Why? Because it prefers the status quo, and exercise is attempting to change that.

The truth is you don't have to accept the status quo.

You can change your brain by changing your mind.

It's mind over matter.

And it's time to set your mind right so you can get moving and let the healing begin.

In this chapter, you will learn the reasons it's hard to exercise and what you can do to overcome the brain's built-in barriers that may be holding you back.

WHY IT'S HARD TO EXERCISE

It was the first day of the new year, and I sat in our home office staring blankly at the computer screen. I had a new fitness goal (to complete a triathlon) but no idea where to start. I needed an action plan. Come to think of it, I needed one for my life too. I opened a browser, and my eyes locked on the search engine. I could feel a quiet resistance building in my body as if it were protesting, "There's no need to change." It was my biological inertia talking, and the discord between my mind and my body warned me that the journey ahead would not be easy.

We all know that the first few steps on any new fitness journey can be difficult. But did you know that the brain is partly to blame? Instead of encouraging us to change, it wants us to stay the same.

Amidst a constantly changing world, the brain strives to keep the body centered around an ideal state — **a homeostatic happy place**. This is your body's comfort zone. Unfortunately, our homeostatic happy place is outdated. Its default settings were established more than a million years ago. Sure, some things are still the same. Body temperature is still ideal at 98.6 degrees Fahrenheit, and the brain and body work together to achieve homeostasis and maintain that temperature. When we get too cold, we shiver, and when we get too hot, we sweat. But the homeostatic control of our **energy balance** is way off. This is especially true when it comes to our hunger dial, which was set to meet the energy demands of a prehistoric time when starvation was a real threat. The **hypothalamus**, one of our most primitive brain regions, controls the hunger dial and dials it up when we move more. This helps prevent starvation, but it also makes it harder for us to lose weight by only exercising.

Although that may sound all fine and good, there is a catch: The lowest setting for our hunger dial is not low but moderate.[1] What does that mean? It means that the brain assumes we are at least moderately active. But most of us are not, and because of this, we end up eating more than we move. **This is why it's so difficult to maintain our weight.** Our modern sedentary lifestyle has effectively broken the brain's energy balance, and for the first time in human history, more people are overweight than underweight.

The good news is that you can restore your brain's energy balance by moving more.

The bad news is that it's harder than it sounds, especially when the mere thought of exercising makes the brain cringe. Why does the brain hate exercising so much? Here are the top *two* reasons and what you can do to overcome them.

Reason 1: The Brain Makes Us Lazy

The number one reason the mere thought of exercising makes the brain cringe is because the brain is lazy. Well, to be fair, it's not lazy per se but conservative.

The brain views all voluntary exercise as an **extravagant expense** and only wants you to move if your life depends on it. To be clear, your life *does* depend on it; however, unlike our prehistoric predecessors who needed to move to survive, our inactivity may take decades to destroy us. Your lazy brain would rather you save your energy for later, when you *really* need it. But let's be honest, there may never be a time in modern-day life when you actually need to move to survive. And that changes everything.

Despite the brain's amazingness, parts of the brain are mere relics of our evolutionary past. Regions like the hypothalamus and its hunger dial were heroes back in the day when food was scarce and we needed to expend tremendous energy to hunt and gather to survive. Just consider the amount of energy expended during a persistent hunt. Anthropologists believe that early humans used this form of hunting to capture their prey by outrunning it.[2] The hunt would begin at the hottest time of the day and would last for hours. This gave us humans an advantage; with less hair, more sweat glands, and greater efficiency of our bipedal movement, we could endure the heat stress longer than most animals.

After hours of pursuit, the animal would eventually collapse from sheer exhaustion, allowing prehistoric hunters like John to capture his prey without a fight. But the marathon chase left John exhausted too. It would take him days to rest and recover before his body would be ready to hunt again.

When not hunting, it was absolutely imperative that John minimize any unnecessary movement to ensure a speedy recovery. John had no problem with this. In fact, he had a reputation for being the "laziest while idle." Although John took tremendous flak for his behavior (especially from the women of his tribe), in the end, everyone benefited from his laziness. You see, John's legs were always well rested for the hunt, making it easier for him to outrun his tribe's next meal.

Ultimately, John's laziness saved his life. It also helped him live long enough to pass on his energy-wise genes to the next generation. Although Darwin might have been confused: "Survival of the fittest . . . and laziest"? It was true. And now all of John's descendants (the John Jr.'s of the world) are blessed with John's energy-wise genes.

Fortunately, John Jr. no longer needs to hunt to survive. Instead, he spends most of his time stuck in lazy mode, and his aptitude for it is remarkable. However, we had best not judge, for we all have some of John's old energy-wise genes in us.

In fact, the laziest parts of our brain are so good at conserving energy that they optimize every step we take. On the fly, our brain sets our stride to be most efficient for the terrain. This is true even for new movements that we've never experienced before, as demonstrated by a study that John Jr. participated in. The researchers outfitted John Jr. with a robotic exoskeleton, which he wore like a brace around his knee, that altered his stride in an unfamiliar way.[3] Within minutes, his lazy brain had already figured out the most efficient way to move to expend the least amount of energy possible. Fascinating, right?

But it can also be very frustrating, especially when you are trying to start a new exercise program. If the mere thought of expending energy makes your brain cringe, you better believe that it'll go to great lengths to stop you from moving, even if your health depends on it.

"Exercise?" questions your lazy brain. "Why would you want to do that? You're tired. Exercising is hard. Do you even have the time to exercise right now?" Its negations are surprisingly relentless and at times almost impossible to ignore, especially when we are stressed out[4] or mentally exhausted.[5]

The most frustrating part is that our brain's lazy appeals endure even when we *want* to exercise. One study used brain recordings like a lie detector test to demonstrate how the brain truly felt when choosing between physical activity and sedentary behavior.[6] John Jr. participated in this study too.

When he arrived at the lab, he was greeted by the researcher. She sat him down in front of a computer screen and gave him the instructions: "For this part of the study, I want you to move your avatar toward the pictures of the physical activities such as walking, running, and biking and away from the pictures of sedentary behaviors such as sitting, lying, and lounging."

John Jr. did as he was told, and the researcher recorded how fast he moved his avatar toward each type of activity. The speed of his movements indicated his conscious preferences. Although John Jr. showed a strong desire to exercise, his brain recordings told a different story. Like a lie detector, his brain's inherent laziness was revealed. Every time he moved his avatar away from the pictures of being sedentary, his brain protested, creating a biological resistance that John Jr. would need to overcome if he was going to successfully stick with his new exercise program.

Logic Overrides Lazy

Fortunately, there is a wiser tale told by a more evolved part of the brain, the **prefrontal cortex (PFC)**. The PFC provides a *rational* rebuttal to the lazy brain's emotional pleas. Rooted in reason and motivated by our long-term goals, the PFC's logic overrides lazy, but it does require some planning on your part.

STEP 1: GET OUT YOUR CALENDAR.

Use a calendar to schedule your exercise appointments ahead of time.

Let me ask you this: Could you imagine working without a calendar? I certainly couldn't. Mine is jam-packed with appointments. Sure, I could fit in an impromptu meeting, but it would take *a lot* of effort.

The problem is that most of us are treating exercise like an impromptu meeting. It's not in our calendar. We are just hoping to fit it in. But there is never enough time, so we never end up doing it.

The solution is simple. Add your workouts to your calendar ahead of time for the next time your lazy brain protests, "Do you even have the time to exercise?" Now, you can wisely reply, "Yes, I've made time for it right here in my calendar."

**STEP 2: MAKE AN EXERCISE PLAN AND PUT IT
IN YOUR CALENDAR.**

We often overlook the fact that it requires willpower to exercise. Game-time decisions drain that willpower, leaving little left over for the workout itself. Plan ahead and save!

What activity will you be doing? When will you do it? Where? And with whom?

One study demonstrated just how effective this simple planning strategy is.[7] They recruited a group of sedentary women who had a new exercise goal. Half of the women were instructed to use a calendar to plan out their workouts ahead of time. The other half were given no instructions. The women with a plan were more likely to achieve their fitness goal more consistently and over a longer period of time than the women without a plan.

Save yourself the time and energy you need to exercise by using a calendar and planning your workouts ahead of time so that when your lazy brain reminds you, "Exercising is hard," you can reply, "Actually, my plan for today's workout is not *that* hard."

Eventually, your lazy brain will realize that it's wasting its own breath and leave you alone.

Reason 2: Exercise Can Be Stressful

The number two reason the mere thought of exercising makes the brain cringe is because exercising can be stressful. But it doesn't have to be *that* bad.

I know you don't *need* any more stress in your life, and neither does your brain. After all, it's working hard to maintain homeostasis, and exercise threatens that. You see, exercise is technically a stressor that pushes your body outside of its comfort zone, and this can make the brain very unhappy indeed.

Here's the scenario: You're vacationing at Yellowstone National Park and are just finishing a delicious picnic when you hear a growl. The sound startles you, activating your **locus coeruleus**. You turn to see a bear, and it's barreling toward you. Your **amygdala** flames with fear, triggering a stress response via the **hypothalamus** that launches its *two* parallel axes:

1. The **SAM**, or sympathetic adrenal medulla, works quickly.
   Using the sympathetic nervous system, it activates the
   adrenal medulla:

   ⇨ **Adrenaline** rushes into the blood.
   ⇨ Fight or flight?
   ⇨ All systems go as you run for your life!

2. The **HPA**, or hypothalamic pituitary adrenal, works more
   gradually. It releases a cascade of hormones from the
   hypothalamus to the pituitary gland, ending at the adrenal
   cortex:

   ⇨ **Cortisol** rushes into the blood.
   ⇨ Stored energy is released from liver and fat cells.
   ⇨ Now your body has the energy it needs to outrun that bear.

Hooray! You've done it. You've outrun the bear. Safe at last. As you
catch your breath, your stress system deactivates. Adrenaline and cortisol
return to baseline, and your body is rightfully returned to its homeostatic
happy place.

Although this bear chase came out of the blue, you'll be ready for it
next time, and herein lies the real purpose of the stress response: to
update the brain's prehistoric settings to match the demands of the current environment. The dynamic up and down of the stress response is
known as **allostasis**, which means stability through change. Allostasis
helps the body adapt and grow and is exactly what we need to become
fitter, stronger, and healthier.

A hard workout is stressful and can induce that same dynamic up and
down of the stress response. By repeating this process over and over,
the brain learns to expect it and helps the body grow stronger and fitter
to meet the new demands of your hard-working muscles. This not only
increases your capacity for exercise but also upgrades your body's comfort zone for other things in life.

However, too much of a good thing is bad. Although we need allostasis
to adapt and grow, too much of it exhausts the body. Resting for recovery
between challenging workouts is absolutely imperative to realize maxi-

mal growth. Otherwise, it will have exactly the opposite effect: **Allostatic load**, which is a fancy way of saying *stress overload*, means you won't get stronger, you'll get weaker. This is the ugly side of stress, and no one needs any more of that in their life.

SLOW AND STEADY WINS THIS RACE

It's easy to get carried away, especially in the beginning when you want results *now!*

Consider this scenario: It's springtime! Hooray! The sun is shining, and the warm weather brings everyone out. They're moving and smiling, fresh and new. But there's some negative too. The winter hibernation has not been good for you. It's time to shape up!

You lace up your running shoes and head out for a jog. The fresh air invigorates you. You run fast and far. The other runners salute you, "Well done, fellow runner. Run strong!"

You do as they say and pick up the pace until you're running with all your might.

Finally, home. Feeling fantastic! You can't wait to run again tomorrow. "Don't break the chain!" you promise yourself, and it's a promise you intend to keep.

The next day your brain protests, "You need to rest." You ignore it and run anyway. The fresh air invigorates you. You run fast and far. More runners salute you, "Well done, fellow runner. Run strong!" You do as they say and pick up the pace until you're running with all your might.

The following day your brain throws down the pain. Aching muscles. Sore feet. Now you're really stuck. You want to run, but you can't.

Days pass before the pain subsides. The setback has set you back. The chain breaks. And so does the promise of a new you. Ugh!

Sound familiar? It does to me. It's how many of my failed attempts at becoming a runner played out. My worst attempt was back in my early twenties. My undergrad roommate, who happened to be a varsity track star, invited me out for a jog. (You can probably see where this is going, but I'll continue anyway.) So, there I was, excited to run with my track star roommate and hoping to finally learn the secret to becoming a runner. We set out together at an easy pace to warm up. It felt great. The other runners saluted us, "Well done, fellow runners. Run strong!" Then she picked up the pace, and my body took a turn for the worse. My breathing sped up to the point of loud and insufferable. My heart pounded vigorously. I couldn't speak. I turned to her in a desperate plea to ease the pace only to find her completely oblivious to my pain, fixated on the horizon, smiling from ear to ear. How could she be enjoying this? It felt like torture to me! Born to run? Not me. I quit.

But I was wrong. And so was my approach.

Finding the "Just Right" Exercise Intensity for You

Do you remember that story about the tortoise and the hare? It's a classic for a reason. Its lesson about going slow and steady is hard to learn. But we need to learn it if we are going to successfully stick with our new exercise program. Our stress system needs us to take a tortoise-like approach with exercise, otherwise things will get very hairy indeed.

A mere fine line separates good stress from bad stress, allostasis from allostatic load. The trick is to get as close as possible to that line without going over it. This maximizes the physical and mental health benefits of exercise while minimizing the risk of injury and pain.

Exercising **too hard** pushes you into allostatic load territory and can weaken you. Exercising **too easy** fails to give you the allostasis that you need to grow stronger and so you stay the same. Exercising at the **"just right"** intensity is where you want to be for optimal growth. Goldilocks approved!

What's your just-right exercise intensity? Actually, it's quite personal. Two people may be exercising at the same intensity: One feels fantastic (my roommate). The other feels terrible (me). Why? Because we differ in our exercise stress tolerance. In my lab, we estimate people's exercise tolerance using an exercise stress test. Here's how it works:

1. Hop on a bike and start pedaling. The intensity is light, and your effort is easy.

2. As the intensity increases, it becomes harder to pedal. Your exercising muscles, which are fueled by oxygen via *aerobic*

metabolism, now need more oxygen than can be delivered. *Anaerobic* metabolism kicks in to cover the shortfall, and this produces lactate.

3. As the intensity increases even more, it becomes even harder to pedal. You feel the burn as you reach your **lactate threshold** — this is your **"just right" intensity**. It's comfortable but challenging. And most importantly, it gives you the allostasis that you need.

4. Every subsequent step-up in intensity is met with more lactate and more stress. Adrenaline and cortisol continue to pour into your bloodstream. Your heart races as you gasp for air.

5. Within minutes you reach your VO_2 max. This is the point at which your oxygen intake plateaus in spite of the increasing intensity. Your body can't keep up with the demand.

6. The test ends almost immediately as your brain forces your body to stop for fear of allostatic load. You've reached your upper limit.

Therefore, your "just right" exercise intensity is at or slightly above your lactate threshold.

Don't have access to a lab? Don't worry. You can estimate your lactate threshold using the **Talk Test**:[8]

Start exercising and ask yourself, "Can I talk comfortably right now?"

If you answer yes, then you are *below* your lactate threshold.

Pick up the pace and ask yourself again, "Can I talk comfortably right now?"

When your answer is no, then you are likely *above* your lactate threshold. Your answer needs to be no at least some of the time to give your body the allostasis it needs to adapt and grow into a healthier you.

In the same way that you can grow your muscular strength by progressively lifting heavier weights, you can expand your exercise stress tolerance by progressively adding intensity and duration to your workouts. In no time, you'll be fitter, stronger, and healthier. And you'll enjoy exercising more too. Why? Because increasing your exercise stress tolerance also increases your enjoyment for exercise.

EXPANDING YOUR ENJOYMENT FOR EXERCISE

It starts in a brain region called the **insula**. The insula stores a homeostatic map of the body. This gives us a sense of who we are, at least physically speaking. Throughout the body, special neurons act like sensors collecting information about the body's current status. This information is sent to the insula and compared to the homeostatic map. Any discrepancy between the two will activate the insula to trigger a stress response, giving rise to feelings of pain and unpleasantness. The insula activity correlates with our rating of perceived exertion (RPE),[9] and therefore your RPE provides a window into how hard your brain thinks your body is working. The accumulation of lactate causes a breach in homeostasis and an RPE rating of 14, which roughly approximates your lactate threshold.[10]

Both RPE and lactate threshold can be used to predict how good or bad exercising will make you feel. This was demonstrated by a study that recruited a group of twelve sedentary men.[11] Liam was one of them. Prior to the actual study, Liam completed an exercise stress test to determine his lactate threshold, and the researchers used the results of that test to set the intensity of his workouts: above or below his lactate threshold. The workouts were completed on separate days, and on both days Liam walked for 20 minutes on a treadmill. The things that differed between the two workouts were the speed and incline of the treadmill, which were adjusted to achieve the target intensities. During each workout, Liam reported on two things:

1. How he felt, using the Feeling Scale from –5 (very bad) to +5 (very good).[12]

2. How hard he thought he was working using the RPE scale below:[13]

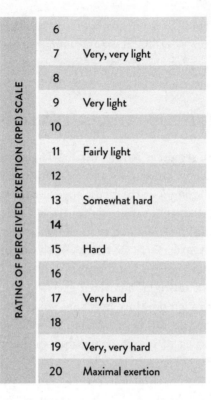

RATING OF PERCEIVED EXERTION (RPE) SCALE	6	
	7	Very, very light
	8	
	9	Very light
	10	
	11	Fairly light
	12	
	13	Somewhat hard
	14	
	15	Hard
	16	
	17	Very hard
	18	
	19	Very, very hard
	20	Maximal exertion

While working out *below* his lactate threshold, Liam's RPE was 10 and he felt good. However, while working out *above* his lactate threshold, his mind and body took a turn for the worse. At the halfway mark, Liam's RPE was 14 and he felt fairly good. But by the end of the workout, his RPE had increased to 17 and he was feeling fairly bad. What happened to him? When exercising above our threshold, lactate accumulates faster than it can be cleared. And for poor Liam, it didn't take long for his lactate levels to soar, leaving him feeling terrible.

Fortunately, you can shift up your lactate threshold with training,[14] which expands your comfort zone for exercising. Therefore, trained individuals have a much more expansive range where exercising feels good.[15, 16] This is why my well-trained roommate was able to enjoy the fast-paced run that was far too stressful for my untrained body. The running pace was still well below her lactate threshold, even though it was well above mine.

If I had only known about the exercise stress response back then, I might have tried a different approach. The real tragedy is that how we feel during the first few workouts of a new program predicts whether we will stick with it over the long term.[17] Running made me feel bad, so I quit.

Born to run? Maybe. But one thing was for sure, I needed to take a slower and steadier approach to have a fighting chance at achieving my goal of becoming a runner.

How to Exercise Right for You

I'd like to take a moment to emphasize that this is *your* fitness journey. You set the intensity of your workouts. Your unique threshold dictates what feels "just right" for *you*. Comparing yourself to others won't help.

If you haven't been moving much lately, walking may already put you over your threshold. That's okay. A baby step around the threshold counts too. Down the driveway. Around the block. Once. Twice. Three times. Start with whatever is comfortably challenging for *you*. I've designed the Wellness Walk (page 18) to help get you started. **Be consistent.** Try for 3 days a week. Put it in your calendar. **Take it slow.** Add a minute or two each week. Then, *gradually* add an extra day, and don't forget to put it in your calendar.

Once you are able to walk continuously for 30 minutes a day, hooray! Now, try picking up the pace, intermittently to start. Eventually, you can replace some of your fast walking with a slow and steady jog. But don't rush your progress. Ever so *gradually*, add more jogging and less walking until you're running for 30 minutes straight. It may take years to get to that point. And that's okay. When you finally arrive and look back to see how far you've come, you'll feel fantastic.

How do I know? This is exactly how I *finally* became a runner. The slow and steady approach worked for me, and I've been running ever since. Over the years, my tolerance for exercise stress has grown to the point that I can now endure high-intensity exercise that puts me well above my lactate threshold, though I try to keep it around **20 percent of my total weekly volume** so as to not overly stress my body.[18] This helps me to harness the healing power of exercise without risking overtraining or injury, unless I'm stressed out. Then the rules change and so must the intensity.

ONE STRESS RESPONSE FOR ALL STRESSORS

There is but one stress response for all stressors. When I say all stressors, I mean *all* stressors, including exercise stress, relationship conflict, abuse of any kind, financial strain, discrimination, work tension, harassment, and racism.

In the same way that moderate-to-vigorous-intensity exercises activate the SAM and HPA axes, so do psychological stressors; however, unlike exercise, psychological stressors tend to be **involuntary** and **long-lasting**, meaning that they are *less* likely to give you the allostasis that you want and *more* likely to give you the allostatic load that you don't want.

If you're here because your mind needs healing, you're probably familiar with chronic stress. At worst, it leaves you feeling **helpless**. And then something very unexpected happens: Instead of fight or flight, stress causes you to **freeze**.

Learned Helplessness and How to Overcome It

"There's nothing I can do to change things, so what's the point in even trying," Leslie thinks to herself before crawling back into bed and burying herself under the covers. Leslie has learned helplessness. How did she get it? By experiencing a stressful situation repeatedly. Over time, Leslie has come to believe that she is unable to control or change her situation, so now she doesn't even try, even when opportunity for change presents itself.

Leslie's human suffering[19] is modeled by the learned helpless paradigm in animal models.[20] The animal lives in a cage where the floor is wired with electricity, and it is repeatedly and uncontrollably shocked at unpredictable times. Then the animal is placed in a shutter box. On one side of the shutter box, the floor is wired with electricity. The animal is placed there, and the shocks continue. On the other side of the shutter box is freedom. If only it could get over to the other side, the shocks would finally cease because that side of the floor is not wired with electricity. Mercifully, there is only a small barrier separating the two sides that the animal could easily get over. But it doesn't even try. Why not? Because it's lived with this uncontrollable stressor for so long that it has come to believe that there is nothing it can do to stop the pain. So, the animal, frozen with helplessness, stays put, enduring the pain. Stuck. Full stop. Hesitant to begin again.

Chronic stress can make any situation seem unsurmountable because it fosters a mindset of hopelessness that gives way to your resignation, like Leslie's mantra: "There's nothing I can do to change things, so what's the point in even trying?" But is her mantra actually true? Part of the healing power of exercise is that it helps keep hope alive. It helped to keep hope alive in me. Of course, exercising will not change another person's maltreatment of you, nor will it remove the systematic social barriers that may be holding you down. But it can create the momentum that you need to get unstuck from your mindset of hopelessness[21] so that at least you'll have a fighting chance when the opportunity presents itself. Although animals exposed to uncontrollable stressors will learn helplessness, the runners among them (who have access to a running wheel) are less likely to freeze[22] and continue to fight for the freedom that they deserve.

Exercise Restores Hope as We Move Through Difficult Transitions

Regular exercise tones the stress response, making us less reactive to psychological stressors,[23, 24] and this promotes optimism, even amidst the most seemingly uncontrollable situations.[25]

One of the most devastating consequences of chronic stress is that it damages stress's off switch.[26, 27] This makes the body **stress resistant**, allowing cortisol to rise to uncontrollably high levels that damage the body[28] and mind.[29]

Exercise protects the brain from the damaging effects of chronic stress by supplying it with a dose of **brain-derived neurotrophic factor (BDNF)**.[30, 31] BDNF acts like a fertilizer that promotes the growth, function, and survival of brain cells, including those that turn off the stress response. Immediately after exercising, our brain cells are bathed in BDNF, which protects those cells against the toxic effects of high stress. Therefore, we can use exercise to fix our stress off switch. In those quiet moments following a workout, our stress system turns off, not just for exercise but for other stressors in our life as well.[32] And in those moments of peace, there is a glimmer of light from which hope springs.

However, there is one important caveat to using exercise to fix your stress off switch, and it comes back to the fact that there is only one stress system for all stressors. If you exercise too intensively, it can add extra burden to your already stressed-out system, weakening your body rather than strengthening it. This is why people experiencing chronic life stress take longer to recover from intense exercise.[33, 34] It's also why people who are feeling overly anxious don't get the same training benefits from an intense exercise program as those who are less anxious, as we've shown in my lab.[35]

The bottom line: Ease off on exercise intensity until those stressed-out, anxious feelings subside. Don't worry, lighter workouts can give you the BDNF you need to protect you brain from stress.[36] And once your brain cells are bathed in that supportive substance, you can begin to move through your difficult transition and into a better life.

HOW TO EXERCISE FOR A FRESH START

So how do you overcome the brain's disdain for exercise stress? The solution is simple: Take it slow and steady. The Fresh Start Workout on page 18 will help to get you started. Use the Wellness Walk and Opener to prime your brain and body for change.

Of course, there will be days when you need a little extra help to get going. What then? Throw on your favorite tunes. This is John Jr.'s go-to. He loves listening to music while he runs because it distracts him and puts him in a good mood. He was also pleasantly surprised to learn that **music makes exercising feel less effortful**. This is something he learned after participating in a study where he ran in synchrony to music with a prominent and consistent beat.[37] For this study, John Jr. visited the lab three times. Each time, he ran on a treadmill at the same fast speed until he was exhausted. The visits were identical except for what he listened to:

VISIT 1: Motivation music with a prominent and consistent beat.

VISIT 2: A metronome with the same prominent and consistent beat.

VISIT 3: Nothing.

John Jr. ran longer and with a more consistent pace while listening to music or the metronome than while listening to nothing. The consistent beat made it easier for him to move. On top of that, when he was listening to music, running felt less effortful, especially at the start of his workout.

TIP: Synchronize your movements to motivational music with a strong and consistent beat to boost your efficiency, ease, and enjoyment of exercising.

An Energy Balance Trick

For those days when you need an even bigger boost, another way to reduce your perceived effort while exercising is to remind your lazy brain that resources are plenty. Remember, the brain evolved at a time when food was scarce, and it may need a caloric boost before being convinced to move. A sugary drink can help. The trick? You don't actually have to drink it. Just swish it in your mouth and spit it out. The mere presence of sugar in your mouth is enough to reassure your lazy brain that resources are plenty.[38] However, the drink must contain real sugar; artificial sweeteners won't work.

BEGINNING AGAIN

Heeding my own advice, over the first few months of the new year, I slowly and steadily strengthened my body, and it healed my mind. By spring, I was strong enough to leave my unhealthy marriage. By summer, I was fit enough to achieve my fitness goal and complete my first triathlon. Get this — I took home the silver medal! Woohoo! I mean, to be sure, it was just a low-key try-a-tri, but still. It was the win I so desperately needed and a good sign to let me know I was on the right track. In big bold letters that sign read: **Keep moving!**

The Fresh Start Workout

REFERENCE: Chapter 1   **NEURO FIX:** Tone the stress system
MINDSET: Slow and steady   **LEVEL:** Beginner

MON	TUES	WED	THURS	FRI	SAT	SUN
Wellness Walk	Opener	Wellness Walk		Wellness Walk	Opener	

WELLNESS WALK
Walk for 10 minutes at a comfortable, easy pace.

Ready to take the next step? Increase walk time by 2 minutes each week. After a few weeks, add intensity to one or two of your weekly walks. For example, 3 minutes of easy walking followed by 1 minute of brisk walking and repeat that four times.

OPENER
Warm up with a 5-minute Wellness Walk, then complete exercises 1 to 6 for the prescribed repetitions. Take a 2-minute rest break. Repeat.

ORDER	EXERCISE	REPETITIONS	PICTURED
1	Arm Swings (up and down)	10 reps	Page 168
2	Arm Swings (across the body)	10 reps	Page 168
3	Hip Twists	10 reps per side	Page 177
4	Knee Tucks	10 reps per side	Page 179
5	Butt Kicks	10 reps per side	Page 170
6	Crossovers	10 reps per side	Page 172
	Rest	2 minutes	

Ready to take the next step? Increase your repetitions to 15 reps. Repeat the exercises a third time.

MOVE AWAY FROM
ANXIETY AND PAIN

It always seems impossible until it's done.

— NELSON MANDELA

OKAY, HERE WE GO, on the cusp of a new fitness journey! Time to move the body and heal the mind to soothe your anxiety, ease your pain, fix your depression, keep you sober, prevent dementia, alleviate your insomnia, find your focus, or optimize your creativity. Sounds great. I'm in!

But wait . . . something's *still* wrong.

You're not quite ready.

Stuck *again*. Full stop. Hesitant to begin again.

What's wrong?

You're afraid, and even before the words are out of your mouth, your mind fills with worry.

Fear.

Panic.

Pain.

Self-doubt.

STOP!

Breathe . . .

And you're back.

Don't worry. You are not alone.

The first few steps on any new fitness journey are the most difficult.

It's one thing to get past the biological resistance of a lazy brain, but it's another thing altogether to get past the psychological resistance of a *fearful* brain.

The secret? You need to get out of your head and into your body.

In this chapter, you will learn how to exercise to soothe your anxious mind.

PARALYZED BY PANIC

The gun went off. Its blast echoed through the air. In an instant, my nervous excitement turned to panic. We hit the water hard. Fast bodies streamed toward the first buoy, and I got caught up in the fury. My body was at its limit: heart pounding, muscles bulging, and mind aflame with fear. I gasped for air but instead gulped a mouthful of green murky water. I thought it was over. I could see the headlines now, tragic yet comical: "Woman drowns in the first 100 yards of her first sprint triathlon." I would be mortified from beyond the grave. Fortunately, that wouldn't be my last breath, but in that moment, it sure felt like it.

This is the power of **anxiety**. It distorts the mind and disables the body. We don't see things as they are; we see them as *we* are. And when the mind is fixed with fear and the brain is infused with adrenaline, the world becomes endowed with danger. The outcome is absolutely destructive and has the potential to derail *everything* we attempt to do.

WHAT IS ANXIETY?

I know you know what anxiety feels like. We all feel it from time to time. It's the brain's natural response to a stressor; and, believe or not, it can help us deal with stressful situations by keeping our mind focused and alert. The problem is that anxiety goes from zero to 100 in seconds. When it gets to 100, we are no longer responding to the situation at hand but to our own feelings of vulnerability. This creates a fearful reaction that is disproportional and overexaggerated. The mind can't focus; it's too worried about what could go wrong. The body can't fight; it's too weak from all the tension and pain. One in three of us will experience anxiety like this at some point in our life.[1] Some of us live like this all the time. The most common anxiety disorders include:

- **Generalized anxiety disorder:** Excessive and exaggerated worry about everyday events for *no apparent reason.*
- **Panic attacks:** A sudden and intense fear that triggers a severe physical reaction when there is *no real danger or threat.*
- **Phobia:** An intense fear or aversion to a specific object or situation that may be *harmless.*
- **Social anxiety:** An intense fear of being negatively judged or scrutinized in a social setting even when it's *not true.*

Worry is our enemy here, and it is causing us to suffer needlessly.

Anxiety and the Amygdala

I love the brain. I really do. But it's not good at regulating fear.

"Uh-oh," cautions the amygdala, "look out! Angry man ahead. Twelve o'clock." There's no real threat, but the amygdala wants you to be ready, just in case. That is its job. Detect threats. Respond with fear.

An overreactive amygdala is the reason we have anxiety. The amygdala reports directly to the hypothalamus, and when it raises a concern, it causes a stress response. Adrenaline and cortisol increase ever so slightly, just enough to notify your body and mind of the potential threat. But when the amygdala becomes overactive, as it does when we're anxious, it stresses out the body and mind, causing more harm than good.

"Oh no!" shouts the amygdala as the angry man moves closer. "Red alert! Red alert! Impending danger!" The warning is relayed to the hypothalamus, which cranks up the stress response full blast. All systems go!

"Ready?" yells the amygdala.

"Ready!" reply your body and mind.

But then . . . nothing happens.

"Where did he go?" asks your mind.

"I don't know," replies your body as it turns around to see the angry man walking away. Still angry but obviously not with you.

The amygdala sheepishly shrugs. "Oops . . . false alarm. Better safe than sorry, right?"

Your body and mind roll their eyes. "Again?" This is the amygdala's fourth false alarm in the last 24 hours. Needless to say, your body and mind are exhausted.

An Anxious Amygdala Is Its Own Worst Enemy

We rely on the amygdala to keep us safe from physical threats, psychological threats, real threats, and even potential threats. Once a threat is detected, the amygdala uses the stress response to warn the body right away without delay. Unfortunately, the amygdala has no way of communicating the *nature* of that threat. The body must trust the amygdala and respond blindly in the same way to all threats, whether they are real or imaginary.

The amygdala is painstakingly diligent. It stays "on" until the threat is gone. That's all fine and good for real threats that actually come and go. Not so good for potential threats that may or may not actually exist.

"If the threat is not real, how does the amygdala know when it's gone?" you ask.

"It doesn't," I reply. And so it stays on. Herein lies the anguish felt by anyone anywhere who's ever experienced anxiety. Take Ada, for example, who lies awake at night worrying about the next day when there is no threat in sight. Her amygdala has wrongly readied her body for battle when what she really needs to do is rest.

An anxious amygdala is its own worst enemy. While Ada's amygdala waits for the potential threat to pass, it keeps her stress system "on" just in case. But this causes more harm than good. It weakens her body to the point of damage, and now she has a *real* threat to contend with. And here's the kicker: Ada's amygdala has completely forgotten that it was the one who created the problem in the first place. Her amygdala sends out a *new* alarm for the stress-induced damage that adds even more stress to her already stressed-out body, and the overabundance of it all damages the body and the mind even more.

An Anxious Amygdala Creates Illusory Threats

Although the amygdala has a blind spot when it comes to its own actions, it is very good at assigning blame to others and even holds a grudge. "Once bitten, twice shy" is the amygdala's guiding principle, and it is constantly on the lookout for any new threats.

A cautious amygdala is roused by any unpleasantry. This is true even for harmless things that just happen to be in the wrong place at the wrong time. The scary thing is that the brain can learn to fear anything. And I mean *anything*. Dogs . . . cats . . . spiders . . . snakes . . . dark places . . . thunderstorms . . . high places . . . flying in a plane . . . riding on a train . . . confined spaces . . . eating in public places . . . using a public restroom . . . being in a crowd. Even exercise.

Although some phobias can run in families (suggesting a genetic link), most are learned through experience. The first study to demonstrate how phobias are formed dates back to the 1920s, when an American psychologist named John Watson wondered whether he could teach a small child to fear harmless white lab rats.[2] Initially, Little Albert liked the rats and would play with them. To get Albert to fear the rats, Watson made a loud and terrifying noise every time Albert reached out to play with one. Soon, the mere sight of a rat caused Albert to cry in anticipation of that loud and terrifying noise. Eventually, Albert's fear spread to other furry white things including a bunny, cotton wool, even Santa's white fluffy beard (I'm not kidding, they actually tested that).

Poor Little Albert. He was a victim of **fear conditioning**. And so was I. Truth be told, I hated swimming. I have a long and storied history with swimming that built up my aversion for the sport. When I was a small child, my dad enrolled me in swimming lessons and encouraged me to become a lifeguard just like him. I worked hard every summer at the local pool and was on the fast track toward lifeguard status. Then one summer, out of the blue, my family moved to a new city. It was a perfect storm. My new swimming lessons began at 6 a.m. in a cold outdoor pool, and I am not a morning person. My classmates were all friends who grew up together on a competitive swim team. I was the newbie, I did not fit in, and worst of all I was the slowest swimmer by far and the only one who couldn't make the cutoff for the timed swim. It was demoralizing, especially for my teenage self. Every Saturday before class, I was sick with worry. During class, I felt rejected. After class, I felt pathetic. Eventually, the mere thought of swimming caused me so much distress that I quit.

Over the course of that summer, I had inadvertently coactivated my swimming neurons with my fear neurons, resulting in a direct connection between the two. From that point forward, any time my swimming neurons became activated, so too did my amygdala, and the illusory threat of swimming was born.

This is the power of fear conditioning. It piggybacks on a fundamental feature of the brain: Neurons that fire together, wire together. And when the amygdala is involved, it uses fear to fasten those wires tight, thus making fear-learning fast and difficult to forget.

Post-traumatic stress disorder (PTSD) is fear conditioning at its worst. People with PTSD are haunted by flashbacks and nightmares of a traumatic event. The "once bitten, twice shy" principle still applies, but their "bite" was life-threatening and now they are *deathly* afraid of it. What's more, their fear spreads to anything and everything that just happened to be in that wrong place at that wrong time.

Paul has PTSD. His fear stems from his tour in Afghanistan when he got caught in the crossfire. Now he avoids large gatherings that remind him of the war zone.

Unfortunately, Paul is not alone. Anyone who has ever experienced a traumatic event can develop PTSD and become deathly afraid of anything that resembles it. But there's more. The traumatic event has altered the amygdala. It is more cautious now. More diligent. More painstakingly protective. When Paul sees an angry man walking down the street, his amygdala burns with more fear, and it is more likely to stay on high alert even after the man has walked past.[3] His hypervigilant amygdala sends shockwaves through his stress system that are almost too intense to bear. "We need to stay away from here," advises the amygdala. "Better safe than sorry." But the amygdala is wrong again.

EXERCISE FOR RESILIENCY

A curious thing is that not everyone who experiences a traumatic event will develop PTSD, and not everyone who experiences fear will develop an anxiety disorder. What's protecting them? A resilience factor called **neuropeptide Y (NPY)**.[4] Some brains make more of it than others. Nick's brain makes more NPY than Paul's. This makes Nick less fearful when he sees an angry man.[5] Nick is also less susceptible to fear conditioning.[6] And most importantly, although Nick and Paul were together in combat, Nick did not develop PTSD whereas Paul did;[7] NPY protected Nick's brain from the trauma.

"I think I might need more NPY," you admit.

"Me too!" I sympathize. And now, time for some good news. You can make more NPY with exercise. What's the exercise prescription for resiliency? It's *easy*. Hooray! One study recruited twelve young male rowers and tracked changes in their NPY during a 4-week training program.[8] All the exercises were performed at a **low intensity** and included light rowing, cycling, and running, as well as resistance exercises done at about half their max load. The researchers measured NPY before and after a low-intensity aerobic workout and found that, with consistent training, NPY increased immediately after the workout and remained elevated for at least 30 minutes.

However, NPY levels increased only after exercise. There was no change at rest. What this means is that *you actually have to do it*.

"How long did they exercise?" you ask.

"Err . . . to be honest, I'm a little reluctant to say," I admit. "Why? Because it was *really* long, and I don't want to scare you. Keep in mind they were well-trained rowers."

"How long?" you insist.

"Two hours. But . . ." I disclose, then rush to qualify before your anxiety skyrockets to 100, "*you* don't have to exercise for *that* long to get relief."

In my lab, we like to find the path of least resistance, and our research has shown that about **30 minutes of light-to-moderate-intensity exercise three times a week** is enough to soothe your anxious mind (I've got your back).[9] To top it off, the exercisers who benefited the most were the ones who were most anxious. I'm also happy to report that they were less anxious after exercising, and their relief from exercise continued to grow with training. In fact, exercising is so good at soothing anxiety that it not only reduces anxiety symptoms in people with an anxiety disorder,[10] but it also reduces the feelings of anxiety that we all experience from time to time.[11] And to make matters even better, many different modes of exercise can soothe anxiety, including aerobic,[12] resistance,[13] yoga,[14] and tai chi.[15]

Exercise as a Catalyst for Anxiety Therapy

The standard treatment for anxiety disorders is exposure therapy.[16] It attempts to undo fear conditioning by repeatedly exposing you to the feared situation but in a safe space. Although exposure therapy is highly effective, not everyone responds in the same way or at the same rate. Some patients take a really long time before they experience relief, and that's not good. It's best to speed things up, and exercise can help the mind heal faster from fear.[17]

How do you combine exercise with exposure therapy? Go for a Wellness Walk (page 38) immediately after each therapy session. Research suggests that exercising during this time may help extinguish fear faster and reduce any residual fear that lingers.[18] The best part? It doesn't matter how physically active you were in the past. What matters most is how physically active you are now.

Exercise as Exposure Therapy for Anxiety Sensitivity

In addition to the benefits of combining exercise with exposure therapy, exercising itself can be a form of exposure therapy, especially for people with **anxiety sensitivity** — the fear of fear itself.[19] If you thought anxiety was bad, imagine having anxiety about your anxiety. It sounds like a cruel joke, but I'm not kidding. You don't have to have an anxiety disorder to suffer from anxiety sensitivity, although it does put you at risk of developing a disorder, and many people with an anxiety disorder are also anxiety sensitive. Unfortunately, anxiety sensitivity complicates the use of exercise as treatment for anxiety, but, as nature would have it, it is the people with anxiety sensitivity who stand to benefit the most from exercising.

Alexia has anxiety sensitivity and gets anxious whenever she experiences the physical and psychological symptoms of anxiety:

- Heart palpitations make her feel like she is having a heart attack.

- A tight chest makes her feel like she is suffocating.
- An inability to focus makes her feel like she is losing her mind.

Her disproportional and overexaggerated response to these symptoms of anxiety puts her at high risk for panic attacks. Exercise is the medicine Alexia needs. In fact, participating in an exercise program has been shown to be as effective as exercising plus therapy for people with anxiety sensitivity.[20] Yet, Alexia hates exercising because it makes her feel like she's going to die. It rouses the same physical sensations as anxiety, which she dreads. And so Alexia avoids exercising at all costs,[21] and when she's forced to exercise, she keeps her intensity low.[22]

"Some is better than none, right?" Alexia asks with fingers crossed.

"Yes, but you would get substantially more relief by exercising at a higher intensity," I explain, as I sadly watch fear fill Alexia's eyes. You see, Alexia's fear of intense exercise is so strong that the mere thought of it activates her amygdala to launch a stress response in the same way any true threat would. On top of that, her sensitivity to anxiety makes matters even worse, because her amygdala views the stress response as a secondary threat and thus launches a secondary stress response to combat it. It's a vicious cycle that escalates quickly and often ends in a panic attack. This is exactly what happened to me during that sprint swim, and I was afraid it might happen to Alexia right then and there.

Luckily, she kept it together at least long enough for me to share with her some really great research. For people prone to panic attacks, the benefits of higher intensity exercise seem to far outweigh the benefits of light exercise.[23] Why? Because higher intensity exercise is the *exposure therapy they need*. Exercising at a high intensity exposes them to the symptoms they fear the most, including heart palpitations and shortness of breath.

"Is it safe?" Alexia asks.

"Yes!" I respond. In fact, new research shows that people with panic disorder tolerate and benefit from high-intensity interval training (HIIT).[24] The researchers used a low-volume HIIT protocol that consisted of:

- One minute of exercise at a high intensity (hard effort).
- One minute of exercise at a low intensity (easy effort).

- Repeat ten times.

I did the math. That's ten exposure therapy sessions in just 20 minutes.

How's that for time efficiency!

The HIIT protocol was completed every other day over 12 days, and the patient's heart rate during the intense burst ranged from 77 to 95 percent of their maximum, which is considered vigorous. By the end of the 12-day intervention, the patients had completed a grand total of *sixty* exposure therapy sessions. With such an intensive therapy, it should come as no surprise that in just 12 days the patients experienced a 40 percent drop in the severity of their panic attacks. Move the body, heal the mind! Hooray!

However, there is a backstory here and one that was not fully discussed in the paper — but it may be the most important result when applying this research to real life. Here's what you need to know: Eighteen patients with panic disorder expressed interest in being part of the study. They even passed the initial screening. Yet only twelve of them actually started the program. What happened to the other six people? Maybe they wanted to exercise but were too afraid. Stuck. Full stop. Hesitant to begin again. I can only imagine the phone conversation between the researcher and a potential participant named Pauline, who was interested in exercising but too scared to follow through.

"Hello . . . Yes, this is Pauline . . . Yes, I'd love to take part in your research study on exercise . . . Yes, I'm free at that time . . . Oh, you want me to do ten bouts of high-intensity exercise . . . Right from the get-go, really? . . . Hmm . . . I see . . . I think I'll pass. Thank you very much for considering me. I wish you all the best in your research, and please keep me in mind for any future studies that involve less intensive exercise."

I get it. High-intensity exercise is scary for people like Pauline who are prone to panic attacks. But high-intensity exercise is the medicine that she needs.

I thought I might have a solution for Pauline to help her get started. Here's the protocol I suggested (it's also included in the Fearless Workout on page 38):

Start with a 10-minute Wellness Walk at an easy pace. This should ignite your NPY to soothe your anxious amygdala.

Then, pick up the pace with a Fear Buster by doing one all-out burst of hard effort. Go as fast as you can for as long as you can. Try for 20 seconds. This will expose you to the sensations of intense exercise without evoking too much fear.

End by walking to cool down.

Pauline was in! At first, she worked on increasing the duration of her intense burst from 10 to 20 seconds. Then, she added in two 20-second bursts and took as much time as she needed to walk and recover in between. Eventually, she added three bursts, then four, and so on, until she was able to do ten. Now Pauline is really moving, and it doesn't scare her one bit.

HEALTH ANXIETY AND THE FEAR OF PAIN

Although PTSD is commonly associated with combat, sometimes the war is within. When a person experiences a life-threatening medical event, like a heart attack or stroke, he may feel as though his body has betrayed him and fear that it will do it again. It is estimated that approximately 15 percent of heart attack survivors[25] and 25 percent of stroke survivors[26] develop PTSD.

"The treachery! The treason!" exclaims the amygdala. "It's hard to trust the body after such an attack." It's been on high alert ever since the event, vigilantly scanning everything for danger. And when I say everything, I mean *everything,* not just the external world but the internal world too: a racing heart, a tight chest, shortness of breath. All signs of potential danger.

"How did this happen to me?" wonders Carl, who has been anxious ever since his heart attack. Unfortunately, Carl's **health-related PTSD** works in the same way as regular PTSD. He has nightmares about having another heart attack. He even goes out of his way to avoid feeling his heart race, which means he's stopped taking the stairs, gardening, even having sex, and you can bet Carl does not exercise. Sadly, Carl is not alone. Every year about 800,000 Americans have a heart attack, yet only one-third of them follow through with rehabilitation,[27] and those who do still struggle to make exercise a regular part of their daily life.[28]

Like Carl, they are not exercising because they are deathly afraid of it.[29] Carl confesses, "Exercising makes me feel like I'm having another heart attack. I just can't bear it." Unfortunately, Carl's health-related PTSD has put him in *real* danger. His anxiety about his heart is keeping him from getting the exercise he needs, and now he is at greater risk of having another heart attack.[30]

Similar fears consume the 50 million Americans with **chronic pain**.[31] Although they are prescribed exercise for pain management, many don't do it because they are terrified it will worsen their pain.[32] Petra, a patient with chronic pain, describes the internal conflict she feels: "I wanted to play tennis, but I was afraid it was going to hurt me." And it is her fear of pain that makes exercising feel even worse. This was demonstrated by a study that recruited fifty patients with chronic back pain.[33] Petra was one of them. She arrived at the lab and was greeted by the researcher, who sat her down in an exercise machine similar to one you would find at a gym. Petra was instructed to push her leg back and forth against a counterweight as quickly and forcefully as possible until she was exhausted. Although this activity is considered safe and unlikely to cause pain, the researcher led Petra to believe that the exercise might aggravate her back pain with the following instructions: "The exercises may cause a slight but short increase in your back pain, but it will not be harmful." Although the instructions were subtle, they were enough to increase Petra's pain rating by 20 percent. She even moved as if she was in more pain with a tense body that restricted her range of motion, diminished her power output, and exhausted her faster. Nothing had actually changed. But now Petra *believed* that the exercise would be painful, and that was enough to make it so. This is a powerful display of the **nocebo effect**, a negative effect that cannot be attributed to the treatment itself and therefore must be due to the patient's belief in that treatment. Unfortunately, the nocebo effect has been complicating the treatment of anxious patients for centuries.

Both Carl and Petra have fallen victim to the inherent fear that the body is in danger. Fortunately, the body is well equipped to keep us safe from danger, which is the real purpose of **pain**. Like fear, pain is another great teacher; its lessons are learned almost instantaneously and are nearly impossible to forget. While fear helps us steer clear of any potential threats, pain helps us to recognize threats in the first place. But there is a catch: Fear shares its intel with pain, and because of this, fear amplifies the pain we feel. This is why fear exaggerates the physical symptoms of many chronic health conditions, including heart disease and chronic pain. But panic attacks are also common among people with chronic respiratory conditions like **asthma**[34] and **chronic obstructive pulmonary disease** (COPD)[35] who fear suffocation with the mere shortness of breath. People with **irritable bowel syndrome** (IBS) who also suffer from anxiety have more gut-wrenching symptoms.[36] Even the anxiety we all feel from time to time is enough to amplify the pain we feel.

How Fear Amplifies Pain

How does fear amplify pain? The brain is to blame. In fact, without the brain, you would feel no pain, even if your body were broken into a million little pieces. A world without pain? Sounds like a dream! But it's actually a nightmare and one that plays out in the harsh reality of **congenital analgesics**, like Ashlyn Blocker. Born without the ability to feel pain, Ashlyn ran around on a broken ankle for days before anyone noticed. Congenital analgesics lack specialized sensors called nociceptors that inform the brain when the body is damaged. Because of this, Ashlyn's brain had no way of knowing that her ankle was injured, so she continued to use and abuse it until it was nearly damaged beyond repair.

Fortunately, congenital analgesia is a rare condition. Most of us have functional nociceptors that alert the brain when the body is injured, and the pain we feel helps protect the body from damage. For example, a kick to the shin during a soccer match causes us to keel over in agonizing pain. Whack . . . *wait for it* . . . Ouch! Your reaction is delayed, but you're not faking. It just takes time for the nociceptors to send their signal along the long pain fibers that extend from the site of damage, up the spinal cord, and to the brain. Although your leg retracts away from your opponent's foot, this is simply a reflex executed by your spinal cord, and it still takes several seconds before the pain reaches your brain. Once in the brain, the pain signals undergo further refinement by the **neural matrix of pain**. Similar to the sci-fi film *The Matrix*, our pain matrix simulates a reality for us unknowing humans. But do not be mistaken: The pain we feel may seem real, but it only partly reflects reality. The rest is an illusion.

The *realest* part of pain is created by the matrix's **sensory core**, but even this is an abstraction. It contains a distorted map of the body called the **sensory homunculus**, which represents the body by sensitivity rather than size (picture lusciously large lips propped up by little legs). When the body is damaged, the nociceptors at the site of injury send their signal up to their coordinates on the sensory homunculus to inform the brain of the size and scope of the damage.

The most *illusory* part of pain is made up by the matrix's **emotional core**, which consists of three brain regions:

1. Insula, which registers the breach in the homeostasis as *dreadful*.

2. Amygdala, which reacts to the body's damage with *fear*.

3. Dorsal anterior cingulate cortex (dACC), which combines the two to create a total sum of *awfulness*. Then, it does something really tricky. The dACC reaches back down into the body to turn up the nociceptors' pain signal. This causes the sensory homunculus to burn brighter (registering more pain), even though the body's damage has not changed. It's mind over matter, and the illusion is complete.

The emotional core is how fear amplifies pain. It is also the reason you feel more pain if sad at the time of injury[37] or if you think someone has intentionally hurt you.[38] It's also the reason the mere suggestion of pain is enough to increase the pain, as it did for Petra.[39]

How does the fear of pain impact our fitness goals? When we fear something will cause us pain, we avoid it. Although this is an innate and adaptive strategy that keeps us safe, when the fear of pain becomes linked with movement, it can prevent us from getting the exercise we need.

THE RIGHT MINDSET FOR
FEARLESS, PAINLESS MOVEMENT

If fearful thoughts create painful experiences, then by minimizing our fearful thoughts, we can minimize our pain and increase our propensity for movement. Indeed, this is the premise of the **placebo effect**, which describes a treatment that has no medicinal properties but comes with a promise that it will alleviate your pain (and other unwanted symptoms), and it actually does just that.

"Would a placebo have worked for the patients with chronic pain?" you wonder.

"Yes, and it did," I explain. Although Petra was assigned to the nocebo group, other patients were assigned to the placebo group. Instead of being told the exercise might aggravate their pain, the researcher told them this: "The movement will not lead to any increase in your back pain." Amazingly, this subtle reassurance was enough to reduce their pain by 24 percent.[40] The patients in the placebo group even moved as if they were in less pain with a fuller range of motion.

We can use this same approach of mind over matter to reduce the negative effects of anxiety on our body and mind. One study simply altered the instructions that participants received prior to a social stress test by telling them to think about their stress response as a help to performance rather than a hindrance.[41] Typically, this social stress test constricts the blood vessels and restricts blood flow, but the participants who reframed their stress response were immune to those deleterious effects. The test also typically induces a **negativity bias**, where participants get hung up on negative words (such as panicky, insecure, worthless, fear), but the participants who reframed their stress response did not have this negativity bias. What I like most about this study is that the changed mindset was not *overly* positive, just less negative. This is helpful because forcing a positive mindset when it's not authentic can make us feel worse.[42]

Ultimately, changing our mindset about exercise can help us move more effortlessly toward our fitness goals. And it helped me overcome my fear of the dreaded timed swim. Those painful swimming lessons I endured as a teen caused me to fear swimming, and I avoided it for years. That is, until 2015, when my dad died of a sudden heart attack and I began to reflect on the things that he inspired in my life. That's when the failed timed swim and my failure to become a lifeguard like Dad really began to haunt me.

I decided to give swimming another try and signed up for lessons, this time in the evenings and in a heated indoor pool to try to beat the odds. I still was an outcast, with 20 years on my swim mates, but this time I didn't care — that is, until the instructor announced that we'd be doing the timed swim. In that instant, my mind traveled back in time to my 13-year-old-self, and I was shaking in fear. Panic. Pain. Self-doubt. Ahh!

But then something different happened. I reframed my mindset with something a little more positive. My mantra? "I am here. I am ready. And I am not afraid." My stress system was activated, as it should be when engaging in a challenging physical task, but I was not afraid. I sang my mantra over and over in my head while I swam with all my might, and much to my surprise, I completed the timed swim second in my class with minutes to spare.

Later that month, I was serendipitously invited to give a talk on brain health with Mark Tewksbury, Olympic gold medalist in the 100-meter backstroke. Before we went on stage, I told Mark my story. He smiled knowingly and affirmed that it was his reframed mindset that helped him win gold. Like me, Mark had a long and storied history with swimming that was marred by the fear of social rejection. You see, Mark was Canada's first openly gay Olympian; however, it took him years to reveal his secret because he had no idea how people would react, and the uncertainty terrified him. Sadly, many people like Mark avoid sports for fear of discrimination related to their gender identity or sexual orientation, and those who do engage in sports often feel unsafe and hide who they truly are.[43] Tragically, this fear of discrimination, stigmatization, and marginalization is creating health disparities to the point that the American Heart Association has issued an advisory warning that LGBTQ+ people are at an elevated risk of heart disease.[44]

Most LGBTQ+ women are not sufficiently active for good health because they are afraid of the psychological pain they'll endure while exercising.[45] Anyone who's ever experienced body shaming can relate. Our fatphobic society causes many people to develop **social physique anxiety** — an intense distress that one's own body is being negatively judged. My friend Anne suffers from social physique anxiety. By society's standards, Anne is overweight. She wants to exercise. She's even made a plan to do so. Unfortunately, she can't get past her preoccupation that others are judging her weight negatively. She even worries that her workout clothes make her look fat. Her shame is so deep that her original workout plan involved exercising at night so no one would see her. In the end, the mere thought of exercising was too *painful*, and she never even started. Anne's fear of *psychological* pain is similar to Carl and Petra's fear of *physical* pain. In the end, it is the fear of pain, be it psychological or physical, that prevents them all from getting the exercise that they need.

Does Psychological Pain Hurt as Much as Physical Pain?

Remember that old schoolyard saying? *Sticks and stones may break my bones, but words will never hurt me.* It's 100 percent false and almost too easy to disprove. Just think of a time when you were ridiculed by your boss, ignored by a coworker, or overlooked for a promotion. How did you feel? I bet it really hurt! In fact, psychological pain can hurt us as much as, if not more than, physical pain. One study compared the two by asking participants to remember a time they felt socially rejected or physically injured and to write about it in a journal.[46] One woman described a painful breakup: "He told me that he no longer saw any benefit to having me in his life." She also described a terrible rowing accident: "It felt like a thousand nails were being driven into my thighs with every stroke." At the time, both events felt equally painful to her, but in reliving them now, the social rejection pained her more.

To examine the impact of social rejection on the neural pain matrix, researchers have designed a clever, albeit demoralizing, way to induce psychological pain in the lab. It's called Cyberball, a computerized schoolyard game of ball toss.[47] The participant, Angela, is led to believe that she is playing the game with two other participants, David and Troy; but David and Troy are actually in on the experiment. At the start of the game, David throws the ball to Angela, Angela throws the ball to Troy, and Troy throws the ball back to David. This three-way toss continues for three rounds. Then, without warning, David and Troy exclude Angela from the game. Angela is forced to stand there and wait while she watches David and Troy throw the ball back and forth to each other. She calls out to them in frustration, "Come on, guys, pass me the ball!" But they ignore her. Angela is forced to endure this for several more minutes until the experiment ends. Afterward, the researchers explain to Angela that David and Troy were part of the experiment, but the damage had already been done. Being excluded by David and Troy really hurt Angela's feelings so much that it had activated the dACC of her pain matrix. Now, do you remember that really tricky thing the dACC does where it reaches back down into the body to turn up the nociceptors' pain signal? Well, it happens with social pain too, and this is how negative emotional experiences like rejection,[48] grief,[49] and anxiety[50] can cause us physical pain.

GET OUT OF YOUR HEAD AND INTO YOUR BODY

We all can do our part to create safer spaces for everyone to feel comfortable exercising, but there is something you can do for yourself to ease the anxiety. When your head is a mess with anxiety, you have but one choice: You need to get out of your head and into your body. You can do that by paying attention to your breath. I see your skepticism, but I have a little neuroscience to back this up. In one study, researchers recruited twenty-six people who had no experience with meditation or yoga.[51] Over 2 weeks, the participants learned how to pay attention to their breath by becoming aware of the body's position and focusing on the sensation of breathing such as the rise and fall of the belly or the rush of air under the nose. Then, their brains were scanned as they viewed threatening photos while either using attention-to-breath technique or not, and the difference was remarkable. When attending to breath, their amygdala activity decreased, resulting in less fear. But that's not all. Remember, the rational part of the brain, the prefrontal cortex (PFC)? Well, when attending to breath, their PFC activity increased, resulting in less negativity; and the calming messages it sent to the amygdala were enhanced, resulting in more mindfulness.

Another study used the same attention-to-breath technique and found that it reduced pain.[52]

Why is attention-to-breath so effective at resetting an anxious mind? Because paying attention to the breath capitalizes on the fact that the mind can only focus on one thing at a time. Therefore, the more time that the mind spends attending to the body (and its breath), the less time it has to worry.

Although paying attention to breath is a natural part of many different modes of exercise, including yoga,[53] tai chi,[54] and Pilates,[55] you can incorporate attention-to-breath into any movement you make, like walking or running.[56] I've included examples of how to incorporate more attention-to-breath into your strength workouts, like the Mindful Mover exercise on page 38.

Added bonus: People who are more mindful are also more likely to stick with their exercise program.[57] And this brings us to the ultimate truth: For the vast majority of people, exercising is not harmful. Not for Carl or Petra or Anne or me, and it's likely not harmful for you either. In all our cases, exercising would do exactly the opposite of what we fear the most. By exercising, Carl could strengthen his heart, Petra could alleviate her pain, Anne could better manage her weight, and I could reduce my anxiety. And I have. I even used the attention-to-breath technique during that sprint swim I talked about at the beginning of the chapter to reset my mind out of panic and back into the race. For the record, I did successfully complete that race. Hooray!

Aside from my panic attack during that swim, my training had made me stronger than I had been in a long time. Though admittedly I was still very uncertain of what the future would bring (and yes, that uncertainty was maddening), I needed a plan to keep moving me forward.

As fate would have it, there was a plan for me. That previous year I had been working with a coach who had helped to prepare me for the race that morning. She had a plan for me and called me up after the race to tell me all about it. "Hmm . . ." I stalled. "A half Ironman, really?" I had no idea what she was talking about but soon learned that her plan would keep me very busy indeed. To put it into perspective, a half Ironman was more than four times longer than the race I had just finished. Fear! Panic! Pain! Self-doubt! STOP!! Breathe . . . And I'm back. "Um . . . sure," I agreed hesitantly, assuming it would be worth a try. After all, I had nothing to lose but fear.

The Fearless Workout

REFERENCE: Chapter 2
MINDSET: Get out of your head and into your body

NEURO FIX: Soothe an overactive amygdala
LEVEL: Beginner

MON	TUES	WED	THURS	FRI	SAT	SUN
Wellness Walk	Mindful Mover	Wellness Walk + Fear Buster		Wellness Walk + Fear Buster	Opener	

WELLNESS WALK

Walk for 20 minutes at a comfortable, easy pace. During your walk, pay attention to your breath.

THE MINDFUL MOVER

Warm up with a 5-minute Wellness Walk, then complete exercises 1 to 7 for the prescribed repetitions. Take a 2-minute mindful break. Focus on your breathing. Repeat.

ORDER	EXERCISE	REPETITIONS	PICTURED
1	Arm Circles (forward)	10 reps	Page 167
2	Arm Circles (backward)	10 reps	Page 167
3	Straight-Leg Kicks	10 reps per side	Page 196
4	Hip Openers	10 reps per side	Page 177
5	Lateral Step Gathers	10 reps per side	Page 183
6	Heel Walk	10 reps	Page 176
7	Toe Walk	10 reps	Page 200
	Mindful Break	2 minutes	

Ready to take the next step? Increase your repetitions to 15 reps. Repeat the exercises a third time. Or combine the Opener (below) and Mindful Mover into one awesome workout and repeat twice.

FEAR BUSTER

After your Wellness Walk, when you feel ready, set your mind to this: "Activating my stress response helps me adapt." Then pick up the pace. Run as fast as you can for as long as you can. Try for 20 seconds. Then, walk to cool down.

Ready to take the next step? Add another Fear Buster and take as much time as you need between the two. Gradually add more Fear Busters until you are able to do ten.

OPENER

Warm up with a 5-minute Wellness Walk, then complete exercises 1 to 6 for the prescribed repetitions. Take a 2-minute mindful break. Repeat.

ORDER	EXERCISE	REPETITIONS	PICTURED
1	Arm Swings (up and down)	10 reps	Page 168
2	Arm Swings (across the body)	10 reps	Page 168
3	Hip Twists	10 reps per side	Page 177
4	Knee Tucks	10 reps per side	Page 179
5	Butt Kicks	10 reps per side	Page 170
6	Crossovers	10 reps per side	Page 172
	Mindful Break	2 minutes	

Ready to take the next step? Increase your repetitions to 15 reps. Repeat the exercises a third time.

3

MENTAL HEALTH IS
PHYSICAL HEALTH

Never judge another man until you've walked a mile in his shoes.

H OORAY! YOU'VE DONE IT!
You're over the inertia and past the fear.

It turns out exercising is not so bad after all.

But life gets busy, and you don't always have time.

A deadline at work forces you to skip a workout. Then four. Then ten. Months later you wake up with terrible chest pain.

A heart attack? You see the doctor but get a clean bill of health.

Relieved, you head home only to have your symptoms return, now stronger than ever.

Back at the doctor's, she explains, "It's not your heart, but your ~~head~~ brain." Depression? Really? But you're not mentally ill.

"Pressure at work?" she queries.

"Possible," you admit, knowing full well the pressure is real.

"Take two a day," she instructs and hands you a prescription for an antidepressant.

You head home confused but do as she says.

The drugs don't work, and now you are *really* depressed.

You slump down on the couch and turn on the tube.

Hey, is that Michael Phelps? You barely recognize him without his goggles.

But it is him, and he's talking about his mental illness. Depression? Really, him?

Phelps describes his symptoms. They sound a lot like yours.

Swimming helped keep his depression at bay.

Too bad you can't swim.

Fortunately, he explains, all forms of exercise can help.

Hmm . . . where did you put your running shoes?

Found! Back of closet. You lace them up, but your energy is low, so you negotiate with yourself: "Just once around the block. Deal?" Deal.

You make it around easily. You had forgotten how good it feels to exercise.

The next day you do another loop. Then four. Then ten. Months later you wake up feeling great! That's when you realize you must make time for exercise because it is the medicine that you need.

In this chapter, you will learn why drugs don't always work for depression and why exercise does.

WALKING A MILE IN MY SHOES

It was a cold February morning. Half asleep, I pulled up a stool to my mom's breakfast bar. She welcomed me warmly with a fresh cup of hot coffee, and we sat and sipped in silence. I had been seeing her a lot lately, much more than normal, and we had already caught up on the latest goings-on. Every other weekend, my daughter and I would make the 1.5-hour trek to my mom's place so that I had someone to babysit while I spent 4 or more hours grinding it out at the local YMCA. Having been formerly sedentary, I often found myself laughing at the absurdity of what my weekend plans had become. But truthfully, I had grown to love it and hadn't missed a workout yet. That is, until that morning, when I quietly contemplated breaking the chain.

The last 2 months had been hectic. I was teaching three courses, directing my lab, mothering my child, and training for a half Ironman. On top of that, I had just returned from a whirlwind trip to New York to speak at the International Neuropsychological Conference. I presented our latest research on exercise for brain health, but now my brain was fried, and I could feel burnout threatening.

As I sat and sipped my coffee, still hoping to summon its effects, my mind wandered to an earlier time when I was under similar exhaustive pressure. It was another cold winter's day but 7 years prior, and I was 4 months postpartum. I pulled up a stool to the breakfast bar in my house and finally broke the silence to my then-husband. This was supposed to be one of the greatest times in my life, yet it was my scariest. The new and intense stress of motherhood aggravated an invisible demon in my head. To the outside world, I appeared calm and confident, but on the inside, my head ached with frightening thoughts about hurting the people I loved. I knew in my heart I would never act on these thoughts, but why did they keep occurring? And now they were directed toward my newborn baby. My anxiety was so intense, I could barely breathe. While trying to be an effective mother, I was living a nightmare in my head that no one else could see. I was desperate for help.

Through tears of fear and embarrassment, I described the nightmare to my husband, who encouraged me to see our family doctor. She recognized my symptoms immediately and offered a clear diagnosis. I was suffering from obsessive compulsive disorder (OCD), a distressing mental illness characterized by unwanted thoughts and fears that can lead one to do repetitive behaviors. "You mean, other people have this too?" I asked in utter disbelief but no longer feeling alone.

As a neuroscientist sitting in my mom's kitchen, I knew that all forms of mental illness originate from a biological dysfunction. The conference I had just spoken at devoted a whole session to it. Yet, when the illness is playing out in your own mind, it is difficult to dissociate the illusion it creates from the reality you're living, while remembering that it's not your fault but faulty wiring.

It also didn't help that, prior to that point in my life, I had purposely avoided learning about mental illness. Why? One word: hypochondria. For as long as I could remember, I'd been worried sick that I might contract a physical illness and die (I know, how morbid). It all began back in elementary school when a young girl in my class died of meningitis. After that, I assumed every headache would be my last. As a teen, I would get the most intense stomach pains and fear my appendix was going to burst. I insisted my parents take me to the hospital, where we'd wait for hours only to have my pain cease as soon as the doctor was ready to see me. Honestly, I wasn't faking the pain, but I couldn't explain what was going on either. So, in college, when I started learning about the brain, I steered clear of any class about mental illness for fear of losing my mind. I couldn't risk it! And now, despite my naiveté on the topic, I had become a textbook case of OCD. Oh, the irony!

TREATING MENTAL ILLNESS: ISN'T THERE A PILL FOR THAT?

People with mental illness are treated differently, not just from the stigma that is born out of ignorance but from the stigma that is built into our outdated medical practices. Most mood disorders, including depression, anxiety, and OCD, are diagnosed and treated based on their symptoms alone. Although this method can be effective, it is in stark contrast to the way we treat physical illnesses.

Imagine showing up at your doctor's office with unusual chest pain. First, your doctor would run a series of tests to locate the root cause of your symptoms: Is it your heart, your lungs, or even your digestive tract? Then, once the biological problem was identified, the most suitable treatment would be prescribed. For example, a positive test for an ulcer would be treated with ulcer medication and not a beta-blocker. Seems obvious, right?

Yet, showing up at your doctor's office with a depressed mood would not prompt her to run a series of tests to locate the biological cause. Instead, you would likely be handed a prescription for an antidepressant drug, and no further testing would be done.

This is exactly what happened to me back in grad school when my strange thoughts first appeared. I remember sitting in class, worried sick that I might blurt out something profane or accidentally hit one of my colleagues in the face with my water bottle. I know, it sounds crazy. It felt crazy! Clearly, something was not right with my brain. I made an appointment with the school psychiatrist. I was too embarrassed to tell him what was really going on, so I described a toned-down version of my strange thoughts. His diagnosis? Generalized anxiety disorder.

And almost before the words were out of his mouth, he handed me a prescription for an antidepressant. This practice is the norm, making antidepressants like Prozac, Zoloft, and Paxil some of the most widely prescribed drugs on the planet.

Why Overprescribing Antidepressants Is Problematic

Over the past two decades, prescription rates for antidepressant drugs have substantially increased, especially for mild forms of depression that may not even meet clinical criteria.[1] It sends a bleak message that a depressed mood is not normal and must be corrected with medication. But is it true? For some, yes. However, this one-size-fits-all approach to treating mental illness is not good for all. In many cases, antidepressants may cause more harm than good. Consider these three points:

Point 1: A Dire Side Effect in Youth

The most obvious issue with overprescribing antidepressants is that the drugs have nasty side effects and equally nasty withdrawal symptoms. Not everyone reacts to the drugs in the same way, and there is a long laundry list of possible side effects that range from mildly annoying to dangerously severe. The deadliest? Suicide.

"Suicide? Isn't that what antidepressants are supposed to protect against?" you ask.

"It is, and they do," I explain. Unless you're under the age of 25. Tragically, antidepressants can increase suicidal thoughts among the children and teens who take them, and the FDA has issued a black box warning (its most stringent warning) to call attention to this serious and life-threatening risk.[2] Children and teens with severe symptoms may still benefit from the drug in spite of this side effect. But for most cases, especially mild ones, this side effect is far too dire to warrant a prescription.

Point 2: A Bright Side to Being Blue

The most controversial issue with overprescribing antidepressants is that there might be a bright side to being blue that antidepressants negate[3] — although I'm convinced that this is only true for mild forms of depression that are triggered by a specific negative event.

The reality is this: When we are sad, our brain gets really good at zeroing in on negativity. Although this temporarily depresses our mood even more, it can also help us resolve the problem that got us down in the first place.

Dwayne "The Rock" Johnson talks about how he used his depression to come up with a new plan for his life. After college, The Rock's lifelong dream of playing in the NFL ended when he wasn't drafted. He even got cut from the Canadian Football League (yes, that exists). Depressed and directionless, The Rock hid away in his parents' basement for about a month and a half until he figured out what to do with the rest of his life. He describes it as one of his darkest times, but he emerged on the other side striving for success. His advice? If you're going through a hard time, you've got to hold on to that fundamental quality of faith and have faith that on the other side of your pain is something good. The Rock went on to become one of the highest-paid actors.

Point 3: The Drugs Don't Work

The most important issue with overprescribing antidepressants is that the drugs don't work for about one in three people.[4] With approximately 260 million people suffering from depression worldwide,[5] we are talking about 85 million people who diligently take their medication but get no relief.

This was the case for a young woman named Pam, who became suddenly stricken with mood swings, anxiety, and hallucinations that forced her to seek medical help from a series of specialists, all of whom prescribed her an antidepressant. Pam took the pills, but her symptoms persisted, and she suffered for years. When the right diagnostic tests were finally done and Pam got the treatment she needed, her symptoms were alleviated completely. What caused her mental illness? A rare but treatable genetic disease called porphyria.[6] The antidepressants did not work for her because they did not treat the root cause of her mood disorder.

Unfortunately, Pam is not alone. Although her condition is rare, there are other more common disorders that disrupt your mood but don't respond to antidepressants. Like Pam, people with these drug-resistant forms of depression continue to suffer, and some may even consider suicide.

WHY THE DRUGS DON'T WORK

Antidepressant drugs only treat a specific biological dysfunction, namely low **serotonin**. Outdated medical practices assume that low serotonin causes *all* mood disturbances. This is not true, but as of right now, no further testing is done to prove otherwise.

What is serotonin? It's a specialized brain chemical that helps us cope with psychological distress. Serotonin keeps us calm by sending messages across a network of neurons. Here's how it works:

1. Two neurons are separated from each other by a small gap called a **synapse**.

2. Neuron A releases serotonin into the synapse.

3. Serotonin binds to its receptor on Neuron B, which excites it.

4. When more serotonin binds to more receptors, the excitement grows into activation. Only then can Neuron B pass on its calming message to its network of neurons.

5. When serotonin is low, none of that is possible and you are left feeling sad.

Antidepressants increase serotonin by blocking serotonin's transporter, called SERT. SERT reuptakes serotonin from the synapse back into Neuron A. By blocking SERT, antidepressants prevent the reuptake of serotonin, hence the name, **selective serotonin reuptake inhibitors (SSRIs)**. With SSRIs, serotonin has a better chance of binding to its receptor and keeping you calm. However, the reason antidepressants don't work for many people is that their depression is not caused by low serotonin.

If not low serotonin, then what?

An Unexpected Cause of Mental Illness

Surprisingly, it's likely inflammation.

Undoubtedly, you've heard of inflammation. It's what protects the body from infection. Immune cells called **cytokines** detect an injury or infection and sound an alarm. The alarm summons other immune cells to the site, and their influx causes the inflammation that we recognize as redness and swelling of superficial wounds.

However, all parts of the body can inflame, even the brain. And when the brain inflames, it causes **sickness behavior** that makes us feel **exhausted, antisocial,** and **depressed**. Sick at home. Alone in bed. Binge-watching Netflix. Sound familiar? Although no one likes being sick, these behaviors are quite prosocial because they isolate us from others and prevent the spread of infection. It's the brain's version of social distancing and a small price to pay for protecting others.

Once the infection is cleared and your health is restored, you are back to being your happy social self again. However, in some cases, sickness behavior persists long after the infection has been cleared. Where does that leave you? Stuck in a funk, exhausted, antisocial, and depressed for weeks, even months. Something is seriously off with your physical state: Your body is inflamed, your mood is depressed; you're not sick anymore, but you're not well either.

Where Is All That Inflammation Coming From?

It's like death by a thousand cuts, where seemingly minor stressors can play a major role in forecasting your future brain health. The impact of minor stressors on the brain's health was demonstrated by a massive 20-year study that tracked over 800 people between 35 and 85 years old.[7] Participants provided a blood sample to determine how inflamed their bodies were.[8] Then, for 8 consecutive days, they recounted their daily stress and how it made them feel. A day was considered "stressful" if at least one of these seven events had occurred:

1. Having an argument with a family member or friend.

2. Avoiding an argument with a family member or friend.

3. Dealing with a stressor at work or school.

4. Dealing with a stressor at home.

5. Facing discrimination.

6. Supporting a family member or friend experiencing a stressful event.

7. Any other event that was stressful.

People who had more stressful days felt **more depressed**. And everyone found it **harder to be happy** on stressful than non-stressful days. However, people differed in how they **reacted** to stressful versus non-stressful days. This was key, but it's also something you can change with the reframing and attention-to-breath techniques discussed in Chapter 2. Some people reacted with dramatic mood swings, experiencing the lowest of lows on stressful days and the highest of highs on non-stressful days. Others reacted less dramatically. The people with the greatest mood swings had the most inflamed bodies, demonstrating the big impact our emotions can have on our immunity.

And there's more. Ten years later, the researchers followed up with those same people, but this time they asked about their mental health. Those people with the greatest mood swings were more likely to be anxious or depressed 10 years later.[9]

And it gets even worse! A person's mood swings at the start of the study predicted their likelihood of death 20 years later.[10] Death! The message is clear: Don't sweat the small stuff or you won't be around. Period.

SWEATING THE SMALL STUFF: A MODERN-DAY SERIAL KILLER

Stress, anxiety, and worry are all common afflictions of daily life in the modern world. A deadline at work precipitates the all-too-familiar routine: Skip exercise, get takeout, and burn the midnight oil until the job is done. Life is so busy now that no one has time to take care of their health. For the first time in human history, more people are overweight than underweight,[11] one in three are sleep deprived,[12] and 80 percent of Americans are not getting enough exercise.[13, 14] Our modern lifestyle is so bad that it's created a new disease category — so-called **lifestyle diseases** — which include heart disease, obesity, and diabetes. According to the

World Health Organization,[15] these lifestyle diseases are one of the top global health threats.

Let's pause to consider the gravity of this:

Stressed out.

Moody.

Inflamed.

Depressed.

Dead.

The scariest part? It's the ordinary everyday stressors that are making us sick, which means we are all at risk. The timid child who can't find a friend. The college student who is late on yet another assignment. The athlete who is desperate to make the cut but keeps falling short. The adult whose to-do list never seems to end. My hectic schedule. Your work deadlines.

"When will I reach the breaking point?" you wonder.

It could happen any day, though, for most of us, it will most likely happen during a **time of transition**.

- The Rock hit rock bottom after he finished college when his lifelong dream of playing pro football came to an end.
- Phelps felt most worthless post-Olympics, when the thing he had devoted his entire life to had come and gone.
- My colleague who recently retired wonders where he belongs now that he's lost the structure and purpose of his day.

For me, starting college, becoming a mother, and ending my marriage were all critical times of transition. Right on schedule, my strange thoughts first appeared during college and peaked postpartum (similar to postpartum depression). What happened when I ended my marriage? Surprisingly, I was okay. But by that point in my life, I had developed the skills I needed to cope with the daily grind. Exercising was central to my strategy (more on that soon). Yet, it still took me a long time to find my footing. To be completely honest, I am still not 100 percent sure who I am anymore or where I am going, and it's already been 2 years. That's a long time to be stressed out, and it is this chronicity that makes stress a killer.

Sick but Not Sick

To be clear, stress is not an infectious disease, but it can make you sick. How? By tricking the immune system into thinking you're sick when you're not actually sick. It's called a **sterile immune response**.[16] It's sterile because your body is free of any foreign bacteria and viruses, but the immune system still acts like you're infected. Fascinating, right? Here are the five stages to becoming sick with stress.

Stage 1: Stressed-out cells trick the immune system.
The immune system treats the body like a private club. Members only! Every cell is checked to make sure it belongs.

- Body cells give the secret handshake. "Okay, you can stay."
- Foreign cells don't. "Get out!"
- Stressed-out body cells know the secret handshake but are too tense to perform it. "Hey, you! Get out!"

Stage 2: The immune system says, "Fool me once, shame on me; fool me twice, shame on you!"
When the immune system detects one intruder and then another (i.e., two foreign cells, two stressed-out cells, or a combination of the two), it calls for immediate backup:

- Regular immune cells increase inflammation a little.
- Inflammasomes increase inflammation a lot.

Stage 3: The immune system (over)reacts.
Bigger is not always better when it comes to an immune response. Too much inflammation is bad for the body, and the consequences range from trivial to tragic.

- It's why when stress-eating, my lactose-intolerant friends and I find it harder to stomach a tub of ice cream. Stress makes us more sensitive to lactose[17, 18] and other allergens.[19]
- It's why we get sick at the worst possible times. Stress makes us more susceptible to infections.[20]

- It's why a stressful job can increase our risk of inflammatory conditions such as heart disease and stroke.[21]

Stage 4: Brain protection and our sixth sense kick in.
Too much inflammation is bad for the brain too. Just consider the permanent and potentially fatal brain damage caused by a concussion that bruises and inflames it. Fortunately, the brain has the **blood-brain barrier (BBB)** to protect it from an inflamed body. The BBB acts like a border wall. It even has specialized transporters that act like border guards, only permitting certain immune cells to enter and with a strict quota on how many can enter at once.

Although the BBB protects the brain from the body, the brain still needs to know what's going on down there. The **vagus nerve** keeps the brain informed. It's like a sixth sense:

1. Eyes see.

2. Ears hear.

3. Nose smells.

4. Tongue tastes.

5. Fingers touch.

6. Vagus nerve detects.

What does the vagus nerve detect? Increases in inflammation, shifts in stress hormones, even microscopic changes in the diversity of gut microbiota. *Vagus* means wanderer, and this nerve literally wanders from the brainstem through the heart and lungs all the way down to the gut, collecting information along the way and notifying the brain of any unusual activity. The amygdala reacts first, inducing fear and launching a stress response. This makes the vagus nerve the ultimate mind-body connector.

When someone says, **"Trust your gut!"** they are referring to the vagus nerve's keen ability to sense when *something is off* even before you consciously recognize the problem. This advice serves us well unless we are **chronically unwell**; then something is off *all the time*. This causes you to lose your intuitive edge. Instead of being in tune, you feel threatened, think negatively, and act defensively.

Stage 5: The stressed-out immune system makes you depressed.
Eventually the brain inflames. Weak spots around the BBB let cytokines sneak across.[22] Is it dire? No, but it is depressing. When the brain inflames, it metabolizes **tryptophan**, creating a toxic by-product that damages the hippocampus.[23] This makes it harder to turn off the stress response and thus creates even more stressed-out cells and inflammation. Tryptophan is also needed to make **serotonin**. Low tryptophan means low serotonin, and now you're *really* depressed.

"Can't we use antidepressants to treat this part of it?" you wonder.

"Good idea but it's not that simple," I explain. Although antidepressants block SERT, an inflamed brain makes excess SERT,[24] and the drug may not block them all.

Now, you're sick with stress. Stuck in a funk, exhausted, antisocial, and depressed for weeks, even months. Your serotonin is low, but the drugs don't work because they don't fix the root cause of the problem. The root cause of your depression is a stressed-out immune system. If only we could screen and treat for that.

Can We Screen for High Inflammation Prior to Treatment?

Mercifully, we can! Though this next part may depress you even more. Why? Because we've known this for over two decades. Back in 2000, researchers showed that a patient's response to antidepressants could be predicted ahead of time based on how inflamed they were.[25] Since then, more than thirty-five studies have examined this effect. Researchers have even narrowed it down to a particular cytokine that seems to be causing the problem, a pro-inflammatory cytokine called **TNFα**.[26] Yet, to date, depressed patients are not screened to determine how inflamed they are. Instead, they are automatically prescribed an antidepressant drug, then told to wait and see if it works. If one antidepressant drug fails, they are prescribed another. Then another. Some non-responders go through three or more different antidepressants[27] before losing all hope.[28]

Was my OCD caused by inflammation? I will likely never know because, just like everyone else, my inflammation was never tested.

Did antidepressants work for me? To be honest, I never filled the prescription. Despite my naiveté about mental illness, I knew a lot about pharmacology, and I worried that the drug would change my brain in more ways than intended. I say that knowing that not everyone has this luxury of choice. Their symptoms may be too severe, their need for relief too urgent. And let's not forget that antidepressants still work for two out of three people who take them.

HOPE FOR DRUG-RESISTANT NON-RESPONDERS

What if you're one of the people who doesn't respond to antidepressant drugs. Now what? Living with an untreated mental illness is a dangerous game that usually doesn't end well. The Rock's untreated depression caused him to hide out in his parents' basement for over a month. Phelps binge-drank to escape his suicidal thoughts. I focused my obsessive mind on my work. My strange thoughts didn't bother me when I was intensely studying, so that's what I did. When forced to socialize, I, like Phelps, used alcohol to take the edge off. But midway through grad school, I realized I was drinking too much and needed a new approach.

I racked my brain for something I could do that would not cause me more harm than good. Maybe exercise? I had heard about "runner's high," and it seemed worth a try. So, I bought myself a new pair of running shoes and went out for an overly ambitious jog. And (as you know from Chapter 1) by the end of that week, with blistered feet and sore legs, my brain forced me to stop.

Then a friend suggested I try cycling, and that's when the rusty old road bike came into my life. On my first ride, I pedaled about 5 miles up the escarpment. When I finally got to the top, *something was off* but in a good way. My mind was completely quiet. Not one peep! My entire body relaxed under its stillness. I hadn't felt that good in years! Needless to say, I kept riding.

With every ride, my mind quieted ever more until a whole hour would pass without one strange thought. Then, the stillness started following me off my bike. At some point, my strange thoughts vanished completely. Was I finally free from the nightmare in my head? Had exercise cured me? Was that even possible? I had so many questions I needed to answer. That's when I shifted the focus of my research and began intensely studying the effects of exercise on the brain.

EXERCISING FOR MENTAL HEALTH

The first fascinating thing I discovered about the neuroscience of exercise nearly blew my mind! Get this: Exercise rescues happiness in depressed patients. And guess who benefits the most? People with drug-resistant depression! One of the first studies to demonstrate this benefit recruited patients with major depressive disorder who had been taking antidepressants but were not responding. The patients provided a blood sample so researchers could determine how inflamed they were. Then, the patients were assigned to one of two exercise interventions: high-frequency exercise or low-frequency exercise.[29]

1. **The high-frequency group** completed (or exceeded) the recommended physical activity guidelines of 150 minutes of moderate to vigorous aerobic exercise each week, for a total workload of 16 kcal/kg body weight/week.

2. **The low-frequency group** completed only a quarter of the recommended physical activity guidelines each week, for a total workload of 4 kcal/kg body weight/week.

Workouts were done on a treadmill or stationary bike at a self-selected intensity for 12 weeks, and depressive symptoms were assessed at the end of each week. By the end of the 12 weeks, everyone benefited from the exercise, but the inflamed patients benefited the most. Exercise not only reduced their depression symptoms, but it also downgraded the symptoms from moderate to mild — a clinically significant change in symptom severity that was similar to the relief that responders get from antidepressants.[30] The best part? Both the high- and low-frequency exercisers benefited equally.

Exercise versus Antidepressants — Guess Which Wins?

In a head-to-head challenge — exercise versus antidepressants — it's technically a tie, which is pretty amazing when you think about it.[31,32,33] However, in some cases, exercise is the winner.[34] And for some people (including drug-resistant non-responders), exercise works better than antidepressants.[35] For example, depression is very common among heart patients. The American Heart Association has even issued an advisory statement recommending that all heart patients be screened for depression.[36] However, the recommendation is very contentious. Why? Because antidepressants are the first line of treatment for depressed heart patients, but many don't respond. Consider the results from one study that recruited three friends, Eric, Andy, and Charles, all depressed heart patients who were sedentary and not receiving treatment for their depression.[37]

1. Eric was assigned to the **exercise group** and prescribed 30 minutes of supervised aerobic exercise where he walked or jogged on a treadmill at a moderate to vigorous intensity three times a week.

   - The exercise program made Eric feel great, and after the intervention, he was depression-free. In fact, 40 percent of all exercisers in this study were depression-free in the end (compared to only 10 percent in the antidepressant group).

2. Andy was assigned to the **antidepressant group** and prescribed the antidepressant sertraline (aka Zoloft) at a starting dose of one pill a day (50 mg) and increasing to four pills a day (200 mg), if needed.

   - The antidepressant treatment made Andy feel less depression, but he also felt more exhausted and had no sex drive. These side effects were so unpleasant that he almost had to stop treatment altogether. In fact, 20 percent in the antidepressant group reported these adverse side effects (compared to only 2 percent in the exercise group), and two participants had to stop altogether because their side effects were so bad.

3. Charles was assigned to the **control group** and prescribed one placebo pill a day. Charles was convinced he was taking an antidepressant even though his placebo pill had no therapeutic effect. Why did they include this control? To make sure that the actual treatments had a real effect over and above the feel-good

placebo effect one gets from merely believing the treatment is working.

- Although Charles felt slightly better (i.e., the placebo effect), he did not feel as good as the exercisers. Also, neither he nor any other member of the control group were depression-free after the intervention.

Although Eric was the clear winner, after the study was over, Andy and Charles joined him on his weekly walks, and now all three friends are healthier and happier because of it. Win-win-win!

The Anti-Inflammatory Effects of Exercise

How does exercise help mend the hearts and minds of patients like Eric, Andy, and Charles? Exercise is anti-inflammatory and reduces the inflammation that can damage the heart and depress the mood.[38] Exercising muscles release specialized cytokines called **myokines**.[39] Like regular cytokines, myokines sound an alarm, but their message is less alarming and more precautionary. The alarm reads something like this:

Dear Body,
There is no active threat. However, we wanted to let you know that while you are exercising and temporarily outside of your homeostatic happy place, you are slightly more vulnerable to attack.

Yours in good health,
The Myokines

The body heeds the myokines' advice, and as a precaution it releases pro-inflammatory cytokines to protect itself while exercising. As soon as it stops exercising, the body sends in an (anti-inflammatory) cleanup crew to clear away the inflamed mess.[40] This cleanup crew is so thorough that they clear up all the inflammation brought on by exercise and then some. With consistent training, practice makes the cleanup crew perfect, and the body becomes less inflamed.

A less-inflamed body is not only good for the minds of heart patients, but also for anyone suffering from a chronic inflammatory condition, including patients with type 2 diabetes,[41] rheumatoid arthritis,[42] even cancer[43] — all of whom are also at elevated risk of depression.

How to Exercise to Prevent Depression

A less inflamed body also helps protect the body and mind from the daily stressors that can affect us all. My lab demonstrated the protective effect of exercise on stress-induced depression by tracking changes in mental health and inflammation of undergrad students across the last 6 stressful weeks of a semester leading up to their final exams.[44] At the start of the study, none of the students were mentally ill or exercising, and we randomly assigned them to one of three groups:

1. **The control group** remained sedentary for the 6 weeks.

2. **The moderate-intensity continuous training (MICT)** group cycled continuously at a moderate intensity for about 30 minutes three times per week for 6 weeks.

3. **The high-intensity interval training (HIIT)** group cycled for 1 minute at a high intensity followed by 1 minute at a low intensity for a total of 20 minutes three times per week for 6 weeks. The HIIT workouts were slightly shorter than the MICT workouts to match for workload, and both workouts included time to warm up and cool down.

Over the 6 stressful weeks, the control group, who remained sedentary, became so depressed that their symptoms warranted clinical diagnosis. This was shocking, especially considering that none of them had a prior history of mental illness. In contrast, and in spite of being exposed to the same psychological stressors as the controls, the exercise groups were protected. Stress did not induce depression in either the MICT or HIIT groups; however, the students in the MICT group ended up less stressed and less inflamed.

Not only did our study demonstrate how quickly mental health can decline under chronic psychological stress, but it also highlighted how effective exercise is at protecting us from stress-induced depression. Amazing, right?

The Stress-Busting Effects of Exercise

The anti-inflammatory effect is one way that exercise protects us from depression, but exercise does something else to protect us, and it comes back to how we react to everyday stressors.

Remember the sixth sense, the vagus nerve? Well, the vagus nerve does more than give us a gut instinct. It's also part of the **parasympathetic nervous system (PNS)** that determines our reactivity to stressors. Although 80 percent of the messages from the vagus nerve go from the body to the brain, giving rise to the sixth sense, the other 20 percent go from the brain to the body to neutralize stress.

It's the yin to the sympathetic yang. The **sympathetic nervous system (SNS)** dominates during stress; it's always anxious to speed things up and insists you have one of two options: fight or flight. But the PNS knows how to slow things down (rest, digest), and it is especially good at bringing the body back to its homeostatic happy place after a stressful event. To illustrate how the SNS and PNS work together, try this quick experiment. Here's what I want you to do:

1. Review your day. Did anything stressful happen today?

   - An argument with friend
   - A deadline at work
   - Witness or experience racism or discrimination

2. Now, remember how that stressor made you feel:

   - Angry
   - Frustrated
   - Tense

3. Finally, check your body. Are you holding your breath?

Under stress, the SNS dominates, causing us to hold in our breath. A deep exhale activates the PNS, restoring calm. That's why yogic breathing is so relaxing.[45] Stress also makes our heart race by contracting it. The PNS lifts the SNS off the heart so it can relax and pump blood. However, the SNS grows heavier as the stressor intensifies. At some point, the SNS becomes too heavy for the PNS to lift, and the PNS taps out. For example, during an all-out sprint, this is the point of volitional exhaustion when you feel like your heart is about to explode.

Regular exercise strengthens the PNS, and it gains with every workout.[46] Eventually, the PNS can lift heavier and heavier SNS loads. Now, you're physically stronger and can push your body faster and harder than ever before.[47] You're also mentally stronger and less reactive to everyday stressors.[48]

More active.

Less moody.

Less inflamed.

Less depressed.

Finally, you are at the root of the problem.

Let the healing begin!

Exercise is medicine that we all need. And I do mean *all* of us. **Not just drug-resistant non-responders, but responders too.** My brother is a responder who suffers from a severe mood disorder that requires medication. While I was training for my half Ironman, he started lifting heavy weights as an add-on therapy to his antidepressant dose.[49] Exercise makes my brother less reactive to daily stressors and less bothered by the drug's unpleasant side effects. Thanks to exercise, he's thriving now too.

Exercises for Mental Health

A little goes a long way! This is true for both the treatment and prevention of depression.

Exercises for Alleviating Depression

A review[50] of twenty-seven studies with over 1,400 clinically depressed adults revealed antidepressant effects from both aerobic and strength exercise interventions:

AEROBIC EXERCISES
- Most studies included three sessions per week.
- All intensities were beneficial, including light, moderate, and vigorous.
- The duration mattered most. Increasing your workout by just 10 minutes yielded a greater antidepressant effect (though keep in mind that the longest workout tested was 1 hour).

STRENGTH EXERCISES
- Most studies included two or three sessions per week.
- All forms of strength training were beneficial, including weight training, yoga, and tai chi.
- The intensity mattered most. Increasing workout intensity by just 10 percent yielded a greater antidepressant effect.

I've designed the Healer Workout on page 65 to help get you started. It includes tips on how to increase the duration of your aerobic workouts and the intensity of your strength workouts as you become fitter and stronger. You get *bonus points* for exercising outside: Vitamin D, which you can get from the sun, is needed to transform tryptophan into serotonin[51] and levels tend to be lower in those with depression.[52]

Exercises for Preventing Depression

In our stressed-out society, prevention is key, and everyone stands to benefit. Fortunately, all forms of exercise help to keep depression at bay. This was demonstrated by one of the largest health studies ever done.[53] It examined the exercise behavior of over 33,000 healthy men and women with no prior history of mental or physical illness. The researchers asked participants how often they engaged in exercise, how long they exercised on each occasion, and at what intensity. They then followed up with the participants 11 years later to see who became depressed. Here's what they found:

> **Who was most likely to become depressed?** People who were not exercising.
>
> **Who was least likely to become depressed?** People who were exercising for at least 1 hour per week at any intensity. At least 12 percent of new cases of depression could have been prevented if everyone exercised for at least 1 hour a week. There was no added protection for exercising more than 1 hour or at a higher intensity.
>
> **The bottom line:** One hour of exercise a week at any intensity prevents depression. Get in your hour by going for a Blissful Brisk Walk and a Soothing Cycle (page 66). And remember, some exercise is better than none.

WHAT CAN WE DO FOR OUR MENTAL HEALTH IF WE CAN'T EXERCISE?

There may be times when you can't exercise. It happened to me postpartum when I was too tired and too sore to move. That's when my strange thoughts bothered me the most. In fact, I nearly unraveled in my doctor's office when I went to see her. Although I was relieved to have a diagnosis, I was still reluctant to take the antidepressant that she was about to prescribe.

"Would it be possible to treat my symptoms without medication?" I asked anxiously and held my breath.

"Yes, of course!" she assured me, which was followed by my big sigh of relief.

She recommended **cognitive behavioral therapy (CBT)**.

"What's CBT?" I asked.

"It's a way of rewiring your brain," she explained. It turns out that many of my symptoms could be alleviated by fixing my faulty wiring. At some point my brain associated a specific thought (hurting someone I loved) with a specific feeling (anxiety). Whenever that thought crossed my mind, it automatically evoked that feeling.

CBT works a lot like fear conditioning but with two modifications:

1. My "cue" was a thought.

2. My "fear" was any negative emotion, including tension, anger, frustration, anxiety, panic, worthlessness, hopelessness, and depression.

CBT works a lot like exposure therapy in that CBT "exposes" you to your thoughts and teaches you how to shift your mindset. CBT taught me to: Pause. Step back. See my thoughts as options rather than truths. With this new perspective, I started questioning the validity of my strange thoughts and why they made me feel so afraid. My analytical brain loved this approach, and when I was able to start exercising again, I combined CBT with exercise. It improved my mental health even more.[54] I had exercise to thank for quieting my strange thoughts while I was in college. I had CBT to thank for helping me manage my strange thoughts postpartum. But it was the combination of the two that helped me calmly transition out of my unhealthy marriage and into my new life. And with that thought, I was back at Mom's breakfast bar.

A MENTAL HEALTH MODE OF EXERCISE

I took a sip of my coffee. It was cold.

"Heading out soon?" Mom asked innocently.

"Soon," I replied, knowing full well the resistance was real. I checked my phone for my workout plan. Had my coach lost her mind?

It read:

EASY BRICK

3-hour bike followed by 2-hour run

(Practice your transition)

Easy? Really? Just the thought of it made my body tense up. My mind raced too, and it was going down the wrong path. I took a deep breath, hoping to redirect it.

Hmm . . . Maybe I could make it *easier?* Coach didn't specify intensity. How low could I go? Some is better than none, at least when it comes to your mental health.

"A Mental Health Mode of Exercise!" I declared. What does that mean? Permission to play rather than perform. For me, it's putting in the time but taking off the intensity.

For Phelps, it's spending his mornings at the gym after dropping his kids off at school. For The Rock, it's doing something other than football.

And with that thought, I was off the stool and at the gym for my "easier" 5-hour bike ride then a run. How low did I go? Funny thing was that as soon as I started, the movement made me feel so good that I ended up increasing my intensity by one notch. Then four. Then ten.

Months later, after months of training, I arrived at Mont Tremblant for my half Ironman race. My body and mind were stronger than ever, and I felt ready — that is, until I began surveying the seasoned athletes. That's when my self-doubt reared its ugly head, and I doubted whether I was properly equipped. To be sure, I had what I needed to swim, bike, and run, but I didn't have the best gear. I raced that half Ironman in my designer sunglasses on my rusty old road bike. I wore mountain bike shoes that required me to first lace up and then Velcro. Fortunately, it didn't matter. My training had made me strong, and on my rusty old road bike, I overtook men on $10,000 state-of-the-art triathlon bikes. That's when I realized that fancy equipment without proper training is just like an antidepressant for drug-resistant depression: It's just a Band-Aid solution that doesn't make you any better.

Beaming with joy, I crossed the finish line in 5 hours 35 minutes, crushing my goal by nearly half an hour. I caught the announcer's eye and over the loudspeakers he playfully teased: "Jennifer, you look too fresh, sunglasses and all! Ready to do another lap?" I shook my head with a spirited "No way!" But in all seriousness, I knew then and there that I was ready for the ultimate test. A full Ironman.

Starting. Finishing. Stopping. Beginning again.

Up, down, and up again.

This unpredictable journey we call life is best taken one step at a time.

Each step you take moves you toward better health.

Better physical health.

Better mental health.

They really are one and the same.

The Healer Workout

REFERENCE: Chapter 3
MINDSET: Exercise is medicine

NEURO FIX: Heal your inflamed brain
LEVEL: Intermediate

MON	TUES	WED	THURS	FRI	SAT	SUN
Wellness Walk	Uplifter	Blissful Brisk Walk		Soothing Cycle	The Remedy	

WELLNESS WALK
Walk for 30 minutes at a comfortable, easy pace. Pay attention to your breath. Walk outdoors for a healing boost from the sun.

Ready to take the next step? Add 5 minutes of easy walking each week.

UPLIFTER
Warm up with a 5-minute Wellness Walk, then complete exercises 1 to 8 for the prescribed repetitions. Take a 2-minute mindful break. Focus on your breathing. Repeat.

ORDER	EXERCISE	REPETITIONS	PICTURED
1	Front Plank (modified)	30 seconds	Page 175
2	Oblique Twists	10 reps per side	Page 184
3	Superman (alternating)	10 reps per side	Page 197
4	Kneeling Donkey Kicks	10 reps per side	Page 180
5	Sit Stands	10 reps	Page 192
6	Row (supported)	10 reps per side	Page 187
7	Lateral Raises	10 reps	Page 182
8	Single-Leg Balance	30 seconds per side	Page 191
	Mindful Break	2 minutes	

Ready to take the next step? Increase your repetitions to 15 reps and 40 seconds. Repeat the exercises a third time. *Advanced progressions:* 1. Front Plank (modified) to Front Plank; 3. Superman (alternating) to Superman and hold for 5 seconds; 8. Single Leg Balance to Single Leg Balance with eyes closed; add weight or resistance to exercises 4 to 7.

BLISSFUL BRISK WALK

Warm up with a 5-minute Wellness Walk. Then pick up the pace to a brisk walk that is comfortably challenging for you. Hold that pace for 8 minutes, then take a 2-minute Wellness Walk break. Repeat.

Ready to take the next step? Hold the brisk pace for an extra minute each week.

SOOTHING CYCLE

Warm up with 5 minutes of easy riding followed by 30 minutes of steady cycling at a moderate intensity.

Ready to take the next step? Add 5 minutes of steady cycling each week. Include a few hills on your route.

THE REMEDY

Warm up with a 5-minute Wellness Walk, then complete exercises 1 to 8 for the prescribed repetitions. Take a 2-minute mindful break. Focus on your breathing. Repeat.

ORDER	EXERCISE	REPETITIONS	PICTURED
1	Kickouts	10 reps per side	Page 178
2	Side Plank (modified)	30 seconds per side	Page 190
3	Bird Dogs	10 reps per side	Page 169
4	Supine Hip Hold	30 seconds	Page 198
5	Pushups (modified)	10 reps	Page 185
6	Cat Cow	10 reps per movement	Page 171
7	Side-Lying Hip Abduction	10 reps per side	Page 189
8	Side-Lying Hip Adduction	10 reps per side	Page 189
	Mindful Break	2 minutes	

Ready to take the next step? Increase your repetitions to 15 reps and 40 seconds. Repeat the exercises a third time. *Advanced progressions:* 2. Side Plank (modified) to Side Plank; 3. Bird Dog to Bird Dog Holds and hold for 5 seconds; 4. Supine Hip Hold to Single Leg Supine Hip Hold; 5. Pushups (modified) to Pushups; 7. Add weight or resistance; 8. Add weight or resistance.

4

FREE YOURSELF
FROM ADDICTION

Life is like riding a bicycle. To keep your balance you must keep moving.

— ALBERT EINSTEIN

HOORAY! YOU'RE WELL on your way. You've pushed through the inertia and past the fear.

Most of the time exercising feels good.

Sometimes it even feels great.

Then something strange happens.

Concerns start to circulate.

A close friend confronts you. "I'm worried you're becoming addicted."

"To exercise?" you ask, confused. She must be kidding.

She's not.

Drugs are addictive. Alcohol too.

Exercise. Addictive? Then why aren't more people doing it?

You consult an expert, and I explain, "You've probably heard of runner's high. It's drug-like, but it doesn't get you *that* high, and that's what makes exercise fundamentally different from drugs of abuse."

The skeptic remains skeptical. "Aren't you just substituting one addiction for another?" Heck, no!

You see, drugs deplete, disrupt, and damage the brain.

Exercise replenishes, restores, and rebuilds it.

In fact, exercise helps the addict's brain heal faster.

It frees the brain from addiction.

A thirteenth step for sobriety.

~~One we can take together.~~

One we *must* take together.

In this chapter, you will learn how to use the high you get from exercise to free your brain from addiction.

HIGH ON EXERCISE

I was high on life for weeks following my half Ironman race at Mont Tremblant. I had never imagined I could do something so physically and mentally challenging, and now that I had done it, I felt like I could do anything. My newfound sense of assuredness brought ease to every aspect of my life. I was more productive at work, more positive at home. No matter where I was or what I was doing, everything came effortlessly. Who needs drugs when you feel this good!

And to make matters even better, my coach gave me full clearance to exercise just for fun. I took long, leisurely bike rides to beautiful parks for picnics with friends. It was a much-needed change of pace from the intense and structured exercise I had been doing. But most of all, I was relieved that she didn't make me stop exercising altogether, as she had done at the beginning of the year. Counter to popular culture, my coach had me take the entire first week of January off and do no exercise. None. Zero. Zilch. While everyone else was finally getting up off the couch and heading to the gym for their New Year's resolution, I was slumped on my couch for the first time in months, binge-watching Netflix. After months of hard training, this should have come as a welcomed rest. But it wasn't. I was restless, agitated, and outright exhausted. I had to take a Blissful Brisk Walk (page 66) just to clear my head, and that was probably offside. (Don't tell my coach.) Ironically, taking that full week off from exercise was one of the hardest parts of my program, and I was training for an Ironman. Sure, I tend to be overly zealous, but my hunger for exercise that week seemed extreme, even for me.

Was I Becoming Addicted to Exercise?

The truth is, exercising *can* become an addiction, but it's rare. Less than 3 percent of the general population are addicted to exercise.[1,2] That rate is only a few points higher among athletes[3] and only 5 percent among the most tenacious exercisers I know — the CrossFitters — who live and breathe all things CrossFit.[4] So, I figured the likelihood that I was addicted to exercise was low.

And besides, I only had one of the four hallmark symptoms known as the **4 C's of addiction**.[5] Yes, I was _craving_ exercise, but my urge to exercise was not irresistible and so my behavior was not _compulsive_. I had been strictly following the program set out by my coach and hadn't lost _control_ in the amount or frequency that I had been exercising. And my training had not caused any negative _consequences_. The only downside was that I didn't have time to binge-watch Netflix, but I more than made up for that during my rest week.

In reality, my exercise addiction was unlikely[6] and almost too easy to prove wrong. Addictive urges cannot be scheduled, and like most people who are recreationally active, I work a full-time job and must schedule my exercise or it doesn't happen. Furthermore, excessive exercise is only problematic if it results in personal or social harm. No harm, no addiction. In my case, there was no harm. And more to the point, just because I enjoyed exercising and wanted to do it did not make me an addict.

All forms of exercise have the potential to make us feel good. A solo hike in nature. A fun-filled bike ride with friends. A deep dive into a refreshing pool. Or lifting a heavy weight up overhead after a smooth snatch. That's because exercising causes the release of a feel-good neurochemical called dopamine. Exercise increases dopamine 130 percent above baseline,[7] which is comparable to the dopamine released by other naturally rewarding things like food (130 percent)[8] and sex (160 percent).[9]

Importantly, though — and the real reason that it's highly unlikely for me or any other athlete to be truly addicted to exercise — the dopamine released by exercise is significantly less than the dopamine released by alcohol, nicotine, and other drugs of abuse.[10]

Alcohol increases dopamine by 200 percent.

Nicotine increases dopamine by 225 percent.

Cocaine increases dopamine by 350 percent.

Amphetamine increases dopamine by 1100 percent.

Although that may sound like a lot of pleasure, too much dopamine is bad for the brain and can result in serious and potentially fatal brain damage.

THE BRAIN ON DRUGS

Do you remember that commercial from the 1980s? "This is your brain. This is drugs. This is your brain on drugs. Any questions?" In the commercial, your brain, an egg, gets fried in a hot pan representing drugs. Although the commercial is not exactly science, it captures the major impact that drugs have on the brain, especially on the reward system, which really does get cooked.

Technically, drugs and alcohol "cook" the brain's reward system by inundating it with too much dopamine. The brain reacts by imposing tight restrictions: **Less dopamine is produced, and fewer dopamine receptors are made.**[11] This is done to alleviate some of the pressure, but it has some unintended side effects.

For one, the small amount of dopamine left in the addict's brain when sober now has even less of a chance of binding to its receptor. If dopamine can't bind to its receptor, it can't induce pleasure. This is the ultimate killjoy.

At first, naturally rewarding things like food and sex seem very dull. Soon, the drug itself loses potency, and the addict must consume more and more of the drug to get the same high (aka drug **tolerance**).[12] That is why seemingly harmless experimentation can quickly spiral out of control. This is exactly what happened to the football player Brett Favre, who inadvertently became addicted to Vicodin, a synthetic painkiller. His addiction started off with an innocent prescription for real shoulder pain. "One pill a day," advised his doctor. But it didn't take long before that one pill gave him no relief. So, he took two. Then three. Then four. At the peak of his addiction, Favre needed about fifteen pills to feel good. That's half a month's supply in one day.

Things get more difficult the longer the addict abuses, as the brain continues to strip away more and more of its dopamine receptors. Now only supernatural pleasures can give the brain the pleasure it needs to feel good. This is when three of the four C's of addiction arise: *cravings, compulsion* to use, and loss of *control* in the amount and frequency of use.

The brain then changes the way it makes decisions, giving rise to the fourth and final C of addiction: Use despite negative *consequences*. The dopamine-starved brain demands **instant gratification,**[13] almost to the point that it would rather die than wait. It convinces the addict that the immediate benefits of a quick fix outweigh any long-term costs of drug use. This is not true. In reality, the addict risks losing it all. Health . . . relationships . . . finances . . . freedom. Even life itself.

At the peak of his addiction, Favre had been abusing painkillers for years, still chasing a high that he had experienced when his brain was fully loaded with dopamine and its receptors. That high was impossible now in his dopamine-depleted state. Nevertheless, he was obsessed. The drug consumed his every thought; it even began to overshadow his love of football. All he could think about was how to get more pills. Fortunately, Favre was able to get the help he needed. You can too. And exercise can help.

Getting the Addict's Brain to Bounce Back

By some miracle, even the most decimated reward systems can be revived. No need for guilt or shame. All you need to do is *stop using*. Only then can the brain get back to enjoying the simpler things in life.

"Right . . ." replies Mike. "Easier said than done." Mike is a former meth addict who's been there and done that. He describes the process of recovery as a cruel game of *hurry-up-and-wait:* First, you need to *hurry up* and stop using to help spare what little reward system you have left. Then, you need to *wait* until your reward system is rebuilt. Unfortunately, as we just learned, the once-addicted brain hates to wait.

How long does it take for the reward system to recover? Based on animal studies, it takes substantially longer to rebuild the reward system than it did to destroy it. Lab rats that used meth for *1 day* took *1 year* to fully recover.[14] Lab monkeys who used meth for *2 to 4 weeks* took more than *4 years* to fully recover.[15] However, in humans, the recovery time is much more variable. One study tracked sixteen addicts who had been abusing meth for the last year but wanted to quit.[16] Mike was one of them, and after spending 2 weeks detoxing in rehab, Mike signed up for the study, and the researchers followed his recovery over the next 9 months.

Mike and nine other recovering addicts managed to stay sober. Sadly, the other six relapsed, a rate that seems high but is typical. What differentiated those who stayed sober from those who relapsed? Surprisingly, not much. There were no obvious differences in age, years of education, or history of drug abuse. Yet, a key difference was hidden in their brains. All ten of the sober addicts, Mike included, had more dopamine receptors than the six who relapsed. If only there was a way to add more receptors to all recovering addicts' brains. Mercifully, there is a way! Move the body, heal the mind.

HOW TO USE THE PRINCIPLES OF RUNNER'S HIGH TO FREE YOURSELF FROM ADDICTION

Exercise increases dopamine[17] and repopulates dopamine receptors to help the brain heal faster during recovery.[18] Although all forms of exercise can do this, runner's high may do it best. If you're a seasoned runner, you know what I mean. Runner's high makes running feel effortless. My highest highs always come during my longest runs. Just as my body is starting to ache, something magical happens. Instead of more pain, I get pain relief. And with minimal effort, I run farther and faster, and the whole experience feels absolutely divine. What's my secret? It turns out there is an exact science to it. A recipe, if you will, complete with *two* secret ingredients that you can use to free your brain from addiction.

The Secret Recipe for Runner's High

Ingredient 1: Endorphins
Endorphins are the not-so-secret ingredient for runner's high. The secret is in getting the right dose. And that takes effort and a willingness to derive pleasure from pain. Think: No pain, no gain.

The brain is hardwired to tolerate the physical discomfort from exercise. It's another relic from our evolutionary past when survival depended on our ability to run through the pains of starvation and exhaustion to chase down our next meal. Nowadays, when we exert ourselves during exercise, the body taps into that same archaic safeguard and releases its stronger-than-morphine painkillers, like endorphins, which help us endure the physical discomfort. To maximize the endorphins released by exercise, we need to push ourselves hard, but not too hard. One study tracked endorphins released into the bloodstream during a 30-minute cycling session at four different intensities.[19] Here's what they found:

1. **An easy pace,** below the lactate threshold, caused no pain and no endorphin gain.

2. **A tempo pace,** at or slightly above the lactate threshold (aka, your "just right" intensity from Chapter 1), caused little pain and little endorphin gain.

3. **A hard pace,** above the lactate threshold, caused more pain and more endorphin gain. Within just 5 minutes of exercising, endorphin levels began to rise. They reached a fivefold peak just after the workout and remained elevated for 20 minutes longer. **This was the ideal intensity for maximizing endorphins.**

4. **A very hard pace,** near maximum exertion, caused even more pain but no more endorphin gain. Essentially, the body maxed out on its painkillers before reaching its maximal exertion.

The bottom line: To maximize endorphins, you need to exercise hard but not excruciatingly so. Thus, deriving pleasure from pain is not as painful as it may seem.

However, there is one important caveat to this study. When the researchers counted the number of endorphins released during exercise, they only counted the ones circulating in the bloodstream. Although these endorphins help soothe our aching legs and blistered feet, they are far too big to cross the blood-brain barrier. In fact, these endorphins never make it to the brain; therefore, they do not get us high.[20] This important fact was overlooked by scientists for years and posed a major challenge for understanding whether endorphins are a necessary ingredient for runner's high.

It wasn't until 2008, when a groundbreaking study used advanced positron emission tomography (PET) to confirm: **Yes! Endorphins are released in the brain during exercise.**[21] The researchers scanned the brains of experienced runners immediately after 2 hours of endurance running. Much to everyone's delight, the hard run increased the number of endorphins in the brain, a whole lot of them in fact, mainly clustered around the emotional core of the neural matrix of pain (see pages 31–32 in Chapter 2 for more details). The researchers went on to confirm the connection between endorphins and runner's high by revealing that the runners who had the most endorphins around their emotional core experienced the greatest euphoria during their run. Ahh, yes!

And there's more! After completing the half marathon, the runners were also happier. Why were the runners so happy?

"Just happy to be done running?" you tease.

"Maybe," I joke. But there's more to it than just that. And this brings us to the second secret ingredient in runner's high. This one will not only make you happy, but it will literally get you high.

Ingredient 2: Endocannabinoids

The second secret ingredient for runner's high is the real reason those runners felt happier after their run. Although exercising is rarely addictive, runner's high is drug-like, and its effects on the brain are similar to one drug in particular. Can you guess which one? I'll give you a hint: It's related to the mellow euphoria you get from a quick toke.

"Cannabis?" you ask in disbelief.

"Yes!" I confirm. It's surprising but true. Exercising is a lot like marijuana when it comes to its impact on the brain. During exercise, the body increases its natural production of cannabis called **endocannabinoids**.[22] How many ounces of exercise do you need to get high? A recent study weeded that question out for us (pun intended).[23] To **maximize endocannabinoids, you need to exercise at an easy tempo pace**, which is not too hard and, notably, not as hard as you need to maximize endorphins. As I said, deriving pleasure from pain is not as painful as it may seem.

Another great thing about endocannabinoids is that they are small enough to cross the blood-brain barrier,[24] and once in the brain, they report directly to the brain's reward headquarters, located in the

ventral tegmental area. When the endocannabinoids check in here, they trigger the release of dopamine in the **nucleus accumbens** to induce pleasure.

"Ready for the most salacious discovery of all?" I ask.

"Ready!" you exclaim excitedly.

Scientists have recently uncovered something quite seductive: **hedonic hot spots**! These hedonic hot spots are found in the brain's pleasure center. They are aroused by both endocannabinoids and endorphins.[25] When simultaneously aroused, as done during exercise, they induce *explosive* pleasure. Now you got it: runner's high!

But the skeptic sees a problem: "If endorphins and endocannabinoids are maximized at different exercise intensities, how can I maximize both at the same time?"

"Buzzkill!" you think.

But not so fast. There is a way to maximize both.

Mix Ingredients 1 and 2

Like any good baker knows, the method for mixing ingredients is as important as the ingredients themselves. Runner's high is no exception. The secret is that although endorphins rise with a hard pace, they *can* be maximized at a lower intensity — you just have to run longer. A classic study demonstrated this in ten trained athletes who exercised until exhaustion.[26] The athletes exercised at an easy tempo pace, which is ideal for maximizing endocannabinoids. For the first 50 minutes of exercise, endorphin levels remained unchanged, but they rapidly rose to a peak right around the 90-minute mark.

Therefore, the precise prescription for runner's high is . . . (drumroll please). . . a long tempo run. This mode of exercise maximizes both endorphins and endocannabinoids for a supremely hedonic effect.

Runner's High (Light): For the Faint of Heart

If the whole idea of deriving pleasure from pain scares you, don't worry, there are a few workarounds to get the endorphin gain without the pain. One option is to **exercise with others**. Group-based exercises increase your pain tolerance, which is a proxy for endorphins. This was first demonstrated in a group of varsity rowers whose pain tolerance was higher when they rowed together than when they rowed alone.[27] The benefits of exercising with others seem to be less about what you are doing[28] or who you are doing it with[29] and more about **moving together in synchrony**. This may be why CrossFit is so popular. Its intense workouts are juxtaposed with an inclusive community vibe.[30] You sweat and suffer together! Your body and brain get pumped full of endorphins so that, in spite of the grueling workout, you suffer less and enjoy it more.

Still scared? Don't worry, I have another option. In fact, your options are endless. All forms of exercise, regardless of the intensity or duration, have the potential to make you feel good. That's because dopamine is released whenever we *expect* something to be **pleasurable**.[31] Even listening to music increases dopamine.[32] So, instead of trying to make pain your pleasure, throw on your favorite tunes and let the music move you in whatever way feels right. Who knows where the music will take you? Maybe to a CrossFit gym. Maybe not. It doesn't really matter. Just keep moving.

EXERCISE TO SHORTEN THE LONG ROAD TO RECOVERY

When the principles of runner's high are applied to addiction recovery, the effects are incredible. Back in 2014, one research group reviewed twenty-two studies that had examined the use of exercise as treatment for substance use disorders, including alcohol, nicotine, and illicit drugs (heroin and cocaine). They found that exercise increased abstinence rates and eased withdrawal symptoms including anxiety and depression, especially among illicit drug users.[33] Since then, one of the most comprehensive studies on exercise for addiction recovery was conducted.[34] The study followed over 100 former meth addicts during their first year of recovery. Mike's friends, Xavier and Elijah, were part of the study. Both men had abused meth for at least a year before checking themselves into rehab. While at rehab and receiving standard care, the men also received one of two interventions.

Xavier was assigned to the **exercise** intervention, where he exercised for 55 minutes three times a week for 8 weeks. All his workouts were **supervised** and **structured** into four parts:

1. **Warm-up,** 5 minutes: Walk on a treadmill at an easy pace similar to the Wellness Walk on page 85.

2. **Cardio,** 30 minutes: Walk or jog on a treadmill at tempo pace similar in intensity to the Craving Crusher workout on page 86, for optimal dopamine release.

3. **Strength,** 15 minutes: Circuit-type resistance training of all major muscle groups, similar to the Brain Bootcamp on page 85 and Phoenix workouts on pages 86–87.

4. **Cool-down,** 5 minutes: Light stretching and calisthenics.

Elijah was assigned to the **education (control)** intervention, where he completed a supervised and structured education program that met for a similar amount of time as the exercise group. The education program focused on topics related to sobriety, including stress reduction, healthy relationships, and healthy behaviors.

Although both men started the study with depleted dopamine receptors and feeling depressed and anxious, 8 weeks of exercise had a profoundly positive effect on Xavier's brain and mind. The exercise program increased Xavier's **dopamine receptors** by 14 percent, compared to Elijah's increase of only 3 percent.[35]

The exercise program also made Xavier less **depressed and anxious** than Elijah.[36] In fact, Xavier felt great and notably better than some of the other exercisers who attended fewer exercise sessions, suggesting that frequent and consistent exercise is important for mental health during addiction recovery.

Finally, the exercisers were less likely to **relapse** after being discharged than the controls.[37] However, the exercise program only reduced relapse among the **"lighter users"** like Xavier, who had been using meth 18 days or less in the month prior to recovery. The exercise program didn't reduce the risk of relapse in **"heavier users"** like Harry, who had been using meth more than that. Unfortunately, the heavier users were equally likely to relapse as the controls even if they had spent their entire stint in rehab exercising. I find this last result really upsetting and have some ideas on how to improve the exercise intervention to help more heavier users like Harry. But, first let's talk about the positive aspects of this exercise program that really worked.

Three Must-Haves for an Exercise Program for Addiction Recovery

1. **Cardio at a tempo pace** to maximize dopamine release plus **strength exercises** for variety, which aligns well with most addicts' preferences.[38] See the Rebuilder Workout on page 85 for an example.

2. **Early intervention with exercise,** as soon as possible into sobriety.[39]

3. **Structured and supervised exercise program,** as opposed to simply unstructured and unsupervised access to a gym. Many rehab facilities give clients access to a gym. In fact, Xavier and Eric had access to a gym as part of the standard programming at the rehab center, and both men used the gym about 80 minutes per week on top of the time spent in the intervention.[40] Although it is possible this leisure-time activity contributed to Eric's modest gains, the speed of his recovery paled in comparison to the superior benefits Xavier got from the structured and supervised exercise.

And this brings me to how the program could be improved for heavy users.

The Thirteenth Step of Sobriety: More Structured and Supervised Exercise for Heavy Users

What struck me the most about the exercisers who remained sober was their incredible dedication to the program even after they had returned home. For example, Xavier continued to log 4 or more hours of exercise per week during the first month post-discharge.[41] However, not all recovering addicts were able to stick with the exercise, and most of them were heavy users. Harry was one of them.

Why was it so hard for Harry to stick with the exercise program? Because Harry was up against a bigger battle. You see, heavy drug use causes substantial brain damage, especially to the prefrontal cortex.[42] Unfortunately, this part of the brain (the rational part) governs the **impulse control** that we need to suppress drug cravings and the **self-regulation** that we need to stick with an exercise program on our own.

Moreover, returning home from rehab is the worst possible time to stop exercising. Why? Because it's when the brain is the most vulnerable to relapse. Sadly, 50 percent of meth addicts relapse within the first 6 months of recovery.[43] What happens during this time? Drug cravings — not the regular drug cravings that come from depleted dopamine, but the **sneak attack drug cravings** that come from the stronger-than-steel connections that were formed between the drug and its cues. What's a drug cue? It can be *anything*: a person, place, or thing that is typically encountered when the drug is used. It's why most alcoholics can't pass by a bar without craving a drink. Or why some people crave drugs after seeing an old party friend.

To understand how drug cues threaten sobriety, I need to introduce you to another brain chemical called **glutamate (GLU)**.[44] Glutamate is the brain's glue that wires together neurons that fired together, and it acts more like **crazy glue** when connecting a drug with its cues. Every time an addict uses a drug in the presence of its cue, more GLU gets added to the wire, connecting the two until they are practically hardwired. It works in the same way as fear conditioning, but instead of linking fear, you are linking pleasure.

Once linked, anytime the cue is encountered, the drug is expected, and this poses a serious problem when it comes to sobriety. When a cue is present but the drug is not, the brain panics and its **withdrawal symptoms** kick in. This is why many addicts must physically remove themselves from their drug-cue-invested environment to get sober. The sterile and unfamiliar rehab facility does the trick. But as soon as the addict returns home, intense drug cravings threaten their hard-earned sobriety.

What's even worse? The longer they abstain, the stronger those cravings become. In fact, cue-induced drug cravings don't peak until a month into sobriety, and they can linger for 6 months.[45] This is why right after rehab is the worst possible time to stop exercising and why the risk of relapse is so high during the first 6 months of sobriety. Exercising during the early stages of abstinence may reduce the risk of relapse later by helping to weaken those stronger-than-steel connections between the drug and its cues.[46]

A 30-minute bout of moderate to vigorous exercise crushes cravings sixfold and puts a pause on drug cravings for at least 50 minutes afterward.[47] Try the Craving Crusher or Endorphin Elevator workouts on page 86.

Regular exercise crushes cravings even on days when you don't exercise. One study found that just 30 minutes of moderate-intensity exercise three times a week was enough to significantly reduce drug cravings in recovering meth addicts at rest.[48] Fewer cravings were felt after just 6 weeks of exercising, and those cravings continued to be crushed even more during the remaining 6 weeks of the intervention.

So, if we bring this back to the original question: How do we redesign the exercise program to help more heavy users? The solution is simple: **We need to extend the structured and supervised part of the exercise program beyond the rehab facility and into real life.** Grassroots organizations are doing just that, and, not surprisingly, many are founded by recovering addicts-turned-athletes who have experienced the healing power of exercise firsthand. Check out Run for Your Life at New York's Odyssey House, Racing for Recovery out of Ohio, and Back on My Feet from Philadelphia. CrossFit clubs are doing the same.[49] All of these exercise programs are providing the enduring support a recovering addict needs to make a lasting change.

THE BEST DEFENSE IS A GOOD OFFENSE AGAINST DRUG AND ALCOHOL ABUSE

As the saying goes: "Once an addict, always an addict." Now I see some of you are cringing, and I completely understand why. When used to characterize *the person* in recovery, this perspective is more hindrance than help. However, when used to characterize *the brain* of the person in recovery, it serves as an important reminder that a once-addicted brain is always vulnerable to relapse.

We are reminded of this tragic reality every time a high-profile celebrity dies from a drug overdose. Prince . . . Michael Jackson . . . Whitney Houston . . . Philip Seymour Hoffman, to name just a few. In Hoffman's case, he was lucky enough to get sober in his early twenties, and he kept off all drugs and alcohol for more than two decades. Unfortunately, his once-addicted brain was still vulnerable to relapse and, seemingly out of the blue, he died from a drug overdose.

Shortly after the news of Houston's death, Bill O'Reilly went on the *Today Show* and harshly criticized her. In his view, she wanted to die, and there was nothing society could do about it. Although he believes that addiction is a mental illness, he does not believe that addicts are slaves to their addiction: "You don't have free will when you have lung cancer, but you do have free will when you are a crack addict." His contrast between mental and physical diseases reveals how little he knows about the brain damage caused by addiction. Chronic drug abuse strips the addict's brain of free will. Yes, exercise can help restore the brain, but it may never be as strong as when it started. And for this reason, the most sure-fire way to win the war on drugs is through prevention.

Exercise for Addiction Prevention

It turns out that exercise is also one of the most effective ways to protect the most vulnerable from experimenting with drugs. Who are the most vulnerable? Anyone with a reward system, really, but especially teens. It is their rapidly developing brain that puts them at higher risk.[50]

The teen brain undergoes an overhaul of its grey and white matter. Grey matter consists of the neurons and other brain cells. White matter consists of the wires that connect all the grey matter together. Up until puberty, the brain is busy building all the grey matter it will ever need. But it goes way overboard. Only about half of the grey matter made is kept. The rest is cut. **Most cuts are made to the prefrontal cortex**, and so many of its operations are not fully functional during this time, including self-regulation and impulse control, making teens more vulnerable to addiction.

How does the brain decide which bits to keep? By exploring the environment. And the curious teen brain is perfect for the job. During adolescence, some researchers hypothesize that the brain is **dopamine deficient by design** to encourage the teen to seek out rewarding experiences.[51] From an evolutionary perspective, this carefree learning is great for survival, but not so great when drugs are around. This puts **children of addicts** at high risk because their environment may be littered with drugs and alcohol. But on top of that, these children may be at greater risk if they've inherited a faulty set of genes that makes fewer dopamine receptors, thus necessitating their need for supernatural rewards to experience pleasure.[52]

Although social and cultural factors still drive higher addiction rates among boys, girls are closing that gap.[53] (Girls, this is *not* a gap we want to close!) **The female brain is more prone to addiction than the male brain** because there are sex differences in the dopamine reward system whereby female brains are more incentivized for rewarding experiences.[54] As a result, the brain of a teen girl is keen to experiment with drugs and faster to escalate from experimentation to abuse.

Exercise Protects the Most Vulnerable from Addiction

How can we protect the most vulnerable from drug addiction? New research suggests we've been going about it the wrong way.[55] Instead of using the standard antidrug approach, we may be better off teaching our youth how to live a healthy life that centers on being physically active. One study compared the effectiveness of the two approaches in over 4,000 students in the sixth grade from twenty different middle schools in Rhode Island. The students were randomly assigned to one of two interventions:

1. **Standard substance prevention program** that focused on preventing smoking and alcohol use.

2. **Energy balance program** that focused on promoting physical activity and healthy eating while reducing screen time.

Both interventions included five sessions over 3 years that took place during that critical transition period in adolescence during which many teens try smoking or drinking for the first time. The results were unexpected. **The teens in the energy balance program were significantly less likely to try smoking or drinking than the teens in the substance prevention program.**

This study raises critical concerns about the effectiveness of antidrug campaigns, like that previously mentioned commercial from the 1980s where the egg (your brain) gets fried by drugs. Even the researchers of this study were admittedly surprised by the results.

Why wasn't the standard antidrug program as effective? The researchers suggested that the antidrug campaign may have backfired by inadvertently piquing the teens' curiosity about drugs. Ever try to tell your teenager what *not* to do? How'd that go? And therein lies the problem with the standard substance prevention approach. We'd be much better off teaching our teens how to live a healthy life that centers on exercise than telling them what *not* to do.

Why was the energy balance program so effective? Perhaps because the teens in the program were more physically active, which would have given them the dopamine they needed to satisfy their reward system. In general, teens who are more physically active tend to be less likely to experiment with or abuse alcohol and drugs.[56]

Although both boys and girls stand to benefit from exercising, girls stand to benefit more. This is not only because they are biologically predisposed to addiction, but also because they tend to be less physically active — a worrying trend that is seen not only in the United States but across the globe.[57]

Run clubs for girls are doing their part to help keep high-risk youth drug-free. The local run club in my hometown is called FAB — for Fit, Active, and Beautiful. FAB is not an addiction-prevention program per se, but it uses sports to help young girls develop the skills and self-confidence they need to make empowered decisions. One of my graduate students is a volunteer coach. She helps train the girls, 11 to 14 years old, as they learn to run their first 5K. The girls work together toward their new fitness goal, not only to increase their physical fitness, but also to gain the mental toughness they need to navigate through one of the most vulnerable times of their lives.

BIKING FROM MY ADDICTION

I really wish I had a run club when I was a young girl. Instead, my dopamine-depleted brain forced me to seek rewards elsewhere and not always in the best of places.

Now, I'm going to admit something that I'm not proud of. Back in my sedentary days, I was a smoker. I know, gasp! My dad smoked, and I idolized him. Coincidently, the summer I quit swimming was the same summer I started smoking. My friends and I were only experimenting, but it didn't take long before I was hooked.

I consider myself relentless, but it still took me three attempts to quit. Unfortunately, this is the norm. Half of smokers who quit relapse within the first year.[58] During my first two attempts, I replaced my nicotine-induced dopamine rush with food. Chocolate cake, strawberry ice cream, and triple-crème Brie de Meaux — all the yummy fatty food you can imagine. Guess what happened? Obviously, that was not healthy either. In fact, overeating can hijack the reward system in a similar way as drugs and can lead to food addiction.[59] So, essentially, I *was* just replacing one addiction for another.

I eventually returned to my healthier eating habits and lost the weight, but whenever I faced a stressful situation (my cue), I craved cigarettes.[60] "What's the harm in just one drag?" my brain begged. But after a few small slips, those stronger-than-steel connections were reinstated, causing me to have a full-blown relapse.

Fortunately, the third time was a charm! It happened when I was in graduate school. Coincidentally, I had just acquired that rusty old road bike, and instead of replacing my depleted dopamine with drugs, alcohol, or food, I replaced it with exercise. And it worked! Of course, it would have been much better if I had started earlier and prevented my addiction altogether. But better late than never.

The Rebuilder Workout

REFERENCE: Chapter 4
MINDSET: Structure and support

NEURO FIX: Give the brain the
reward it seeks
LEVEL: Intermediate

MON	TUES	WED	THURS	FRI	SAT	SUN
Wellness Walk	Brain Boot-camp	Craving Crusher	The Neuro Fix	Endorphin Elevator	Phoenix	

WELLNESS WALK

Walk for 30 minutes at a comfortable, easy pace. Listen to music and walk with friends for an extra neuro boost.

BRAIN BOOTCAMP

Warm up with a 5-minute Wellness Walk, then complete exercises 1 to 4 in Circuit #1 for the prescribed repetitions. Take a 2-minute mindful break. Focus on your breathing. Repeat. Then move on to Circuit #2. Repeat.

Circuit #1

ORDER	EXERCISE	REPETITIONS	PICTURED
1	Pushups	10 reps	Page 185
2	Row (single arm)	10 reps per side	Page 187
3	Bird Dogs (5-second holds)	10 reps per side	Page 169
4	Bicycles	10 reps per side	Page 169
	Mindful Break	2 minutes	

Circuit #2

ORDER	EXERCISE	REPETITIONS	PICTURED
1	Split Squats	10 reps per side	Page 194
2	Supine Hip Lifts	10 reps	Page 198
3	Mountain Climbers	10 reps per side	Page 184
4	Side Plank	30 seconds per side	Page 190
	Mindful Break	2 minutes	

Ready to take the next step? Increase your repetitions to 15 reps and 40 seconds. Repeat the exercises a third time.

CRAVING CRUSHER

Warm up with a 5-minute Wellness Walk, then pick up the pace until it is comfortably challenging for you (brisk walk or easy jog). Hold that pace for 60 seconds, then take a 2-minute Wellness Walk break. Repeat five times. Cool down with a 10-minute Wellness Walk.

Ready to take the next step? Repeat six times and add another repeat each week.

THE NEURO FIX

Do it anywhere anytime you need it: Warm up with a 5-minute Wellness Walk, then complete exercises 1 to 4. Work as hard as you can. Repeat.

ORDER	EXERCISE	REPETITIONS	PICTURED
1	Jumping Jacks	30 seconds	Page 178
2	Mountain Climbers	30 seconds	Page 184
3	Skaters	30 seconds	Page 193
4	High Knees	30 seconds	Page 176

ENDORPHIN ELEVATOR

Take the stairs! Warm up with a 10-minute Wellness Walk. Then climb a set of stairs for 60 seconds, walk down, rest for 30 seconds. Repeat five times. Cool down with a 10-minute Wellness Walk.

Ready to take the next step? Add an extra 60-second stair climb every week.

PHOENIX

Warm up with a 5-minute Wellness Walk, then complete exercises 1 to 4 in Circuit #1 for the prescribed repetitions. Take a 2-minute mindful break. Focus on your breathing. Repeat. Then move on to Circuit #2. Repeat.

Circuit #1

ORDER	EXERCISE	REPETITIONS	PICTURED
1	Shoulder Presses (with Bicep Curl)	10 reps	Page 188
2	Reverse Flies	10 reps	Page 186
3	Kneeling Woodchoppers	10 reps per side	Page 181
4	Dead Bugs	10 reps per side	Page 173
	Mindful Break	2 minutes	

Circuit #2

ORDER	EXERCISE	REPETITIONS	PICTURED
1	Sumo Squats	10 reps	Page 197
2	Side-Lying Hip Abduction	10 reps per side	Page 189
3	Side-Lying Hip Adduction	10 reps per side	Page 189
4	Front Plank	30 seconds per side	Page 175
	Mindful Break	2 minutes	

Ready to take the next step? Increase your repetitions to 15 reps and 40 seconds. Repeat the exercises a third time.

5

KEEP YOUR
BRAIN YOUNG

Fun never asks how old you are.

YOU'RE OLDER NOW, but you don't feel your age.

And you don't fit the stereotype: depressed, lonely, physically frail, mentally limited.

No, thanks!

"You seem so young!" friends proclaim.

"What's your secret?" others wonder.

"A walk a day keeps dementia at bay," you say, and then one day one friend listens.

He's an old friend. You went to high school together.

You're the same age, but most people think he's older.

His wife died last year, and he's been lonely ever since.

You were surprised to hear from him. But he trusts you and knows you walk every day.

At his last checkup, his doctor warned that his health was declining too fast.

"No one wants dementia," his doctor cautioned, and recommended exercising.

He meets you at the park, and you start out at your usual pace, but he can't keep up. So, you slow down and suggest, "Once around the park?" He agrees but barely makes it.

The next day, he's back. And he keeps coming back. The following day. And the day after that. And the day after that too. Weeks go by. The seasons change. It's hard to believe it's been a year. "Time flies when you're having fun," you both say in synchrony and laugh.

Now, you're really moving. Covering lots of distance too.

Not just once around the park, or twice, but ten times at a brisk pace.

Soon you'll need to add in hill repeats just to break a sweat.

"Did you hear about the exercise pill?" you ask him, making conversation during one of the walks. You had read about it in the newspaper earlier that morning.

He smiles, takes your hand in his, and confides, "Exercise pill? No, thanks. I'd rather walk with you."

In this chapter, you will learn how stereotypes about aging threaten our brain health. Then, I will give you the CliffsNotes for my master's course in Brain Health and Aging that can be done at any time in your lifetime but preferably before midlife.

STRONGER TOGETHER

"We're all in this together!" I heard someone exclaim during my race at Mont Tremblant, and it has stuck with me ever since. If there is one thing I love about a triathlon, it's the camaraderie. Fast friendships are formed, which means that instead of sweating it out on my own, I am out on an exercise adventure with my new "exercise friends," and it is so much more fun! Two of my new friends had just qualified for the half Ironman world championships in New Zealand, and I wanted to qualify too.

To qualify, I needed to be faster. Only the first and second place finishers were guaranteed a spot. I did the math. The only thing standing between me and my world championship debut was an additional 30 minutes shaved off my finishing time. Was that even possible at my age?

I looked into it and was shocked to learn that the first woman to cross the finish line at Mont Tremblant that year was Mirinda Carfrae, born exactly 13 days before me. Hmm ... maybe it was possible after all. I immediately booked a session with my coach to see if she agreed.

The next qualifying race was at Lake Placid, only 10 weeks away, but my coach thought it was doable and prepared an intensive program to get me in top shape. I trained hard with my new exercise friends by my side, and the time flew by. But as the race neared, my self-doubt reared its ugly head (again) and filled my mind with self-limiting thoughts: "Pushing 40 and trying to qualify for a world championship event in a sport you just joined. Are you out of your mind?" Surely, I was joining too late in the game.

Then I learned about the Iron Nun, Sister Madonna Buder, who was born in St. Louis, Missouri. At the age of 86, she had completed over forty Ironman events — and was preparing for her next. If that isn't inspiring enough, her entry into that race broke the glass ceiling in triathlons and opened a whole new age group for women. Going against her mother's advice to act her age, the Iron Nun subscribes to a different philosophy: Age is a matter of mind. If you don't mind, it doesn't matter. She doesn't notice herself getting older because exercising invigorates her.

WHAT'S YOUR STEREOTYPE ON AGING?

"Getting old sucks," one reader interjects.

Umm . . . okay.

Unfortunately, not everyone subscribes to the Iron Nun's philosophy. To be fair, the reader does have a point. Life can be exhausting. Even depressing. Aging distorts the body and mind. And the media doesn't help either. Showcasing all those beautiful 20-somethings, bouncing around with all that energy. It makes your slog up and over the hill seem extra burdensome. "Do you need a hand?" one of the 20-somethings asks politely. You scowl because it feels like she's mocking you. She's not.

Depressed. Lonely. Physically frail. Mentally limited. Some people embody this stereotype of aging. Where does it come from? The past, when that was all that aging could be. But it's outdated, archaic, and old-fashioned. Just look at those zoomers! They've given aging a facelift. Not only do they look younger than their age; they act younger too. Some seniors are more active now than ever before, and they're healthier for it.

It raises the question: How do today's children view older people? To find out, I conducted a little experiment on my daughter and her friend. I asked them to draw a picture of people who were young and old. I was shocked at what they drew.

For starters, the drawing they showed me was absolutely beautiful, full of exquisite detail.

It depicted the timeline of a woman's life that included four stages: baby . . . child . . . mother . . . grandmother.

The small baby grew and grew and grew until she became a mother. Then, as a grandmother, her stature severely shriveled to the height and weight of a small child. And to make matters even worse, she was carrying a cane. A cane! Clearly, my pro-aging messages were not getting through.

But perhaps my method was flawed. Some researchers suggest that drawings do not fully capture how a child feels about older people.[1] With this in mind, I revised my test. This time, I asked Monica to describe an older person using her own words.

She spoke kindly. "Gentle, social, and smart," she reflected.

"That's my girl!" I cheered proudly and asked, "Who are you thinking of?"

"Grandma," she replied. My heart melted. My darling girl was getting my messages after all. It helped that her grandmother was fit and active. The question remained: Did she feel that way about all older people? I asked again, this time prompting her to think of a random older person. The words came quickly, and in a deep wretched voice she growled, "Cranky. Get off my lawn!" Clearly, I have more work to do.

According to research,[2] most children share my daughter's double standard about aging. They revere and respect older people they know, yet apply a harsh ageist stereotype to strangers.

What this means is that two children may be looking at the same older person. One child sees the person. The other child "sees" the stereotype. And this changes everything. It may seem funny now. You may even laugh out loud and say, "Kids these days!" But your laughter only serves to reinforce the stereotype. At first, stereotypes affect the way the child sees older people. Soon, it will affect the way she treats them.

Eventually, and here's the real kicker, when the child grows old, her harsh views about aging will become her harsh views about herself — a self-fulfilling prophecy. At its worst, the once-child-now-senior typecasts herself as depressed, lonely, physically frail, and mentally limited.[3] Getting old sucks when you see it that way.

Don't Say the D-Word

Dementia (sorry, I had to say it) has become synonymous with aging. People are terrified of it. And for good reason. Alzheimer's disease has the power to strip you of your personal past to the point that you forget who you are. If that wasn't bad enough, the stigma associated with the disease makes you feel even worse. This was so pointedly captured in the movie *Still Alice*, which portrays the unraveling of a woman diagnosed with Alzheimer's disease. Not only must Alice learn to face the devasting symptoms of the disease but also the indignity of her own stigma. At one point, Alice confides, "I wish I had cancer. I wouldn't feel so ashamed." I watched the movie with my mom. We both wept at that part, heartbroken for her.

Although my mom is mentally sharp and physically active, she is terrified of getting dementia. Her brother has early signs of decline, and watching the movie only amplified her concerns. I tried to explain to my mom:

Aging does *not* equal dementia.
And worrying about it does more harm than good.

"It's hard *not* to be afraid of it," she said.

Unfortunately, my mom is not alone. The fear of growing old and becoming senile is a global concern. But it's hard to live your best life now when you're worried that the worst has yet to come. One study demonstrated just how hard it is to think when preoccupied about your waning memory.[4] The study recruited over 100 older adults. Two friends, Patrick and Naveen, were among the participants. Both men were 60, well educated, and in great shape. Neither had any issue with their memory — that is, until that day.

The men arrived at the lab and were greeted by the researcher. "I want you to study these words," she explained, and handed each of them a sheet of paper with thirty words on it. "I'll be testing your memory for these words later."

Patrick and Naveen studied the list of words for 2 minutes. Then, she randomly assigned the men to one of two groups:

1. Patrick was assigned to the **non-threat group**. He was told that the memory test was free of any age bias, and he was not asked his age.

2. Naveen was assigned to the **threat group**. He was told that the memory test was designed to examine age differences between young and old. Then he was asked his age.

   - Why did the researcher do those things? She emphasized *age differences* to remind Naveen that old people have worse memory than young people. She asked *his age* to remind him that he was one of those old people.

The mere thought of being old and senile was enough to impair Naveen's memory, and he recalled fewer words than Patrick. The researcher was not surprised, especially since Naveen was relatively young and highly educated. People like Naveen worry the most about getting dementia. The researcher called him "worried but well" — a term she reserves for older people who are mentally capable but overly self-conscious. "They are so worried about their memory loss," she explained, "that it distracts them from the present moment so much so that they *seem* impaired, even though they are perfectly healthy."

Slowed Down by Stereotype Threats

Stereotype threats can also impact an older adult's physical performance, and it can alter something as fundamental as their **walking speed**. The dominant stereotype is that seniors are slow. Because this opinion is so pervasive, many older adults inadvertently walk slower just to match this lower expectation. Patrick and Naveen took part in another study that evaluated this.[5] The men were greeted and instructed to walk as fast as they could down a 45-meter hallway. Patrick and Naveen walked down the hallway at the same speed. Then, each man sat down in front of a computer. A series of words were flashed on the screen. The men were told to indicate whether the "flash" appeared above or below a central point. What they didn't realize was that those "flashes" were actually words, presented too fast to be read consciously yet slow enough to be registered by the brain. The two men were flashed different words.

1. Patrick was flashed **age-positive words**: wise, astute, and accomplished, which *decreased* his stereotype threat.

2. Naveen was flashed **age-negative words**: senile, dependent, and diseased, which *increased* his stereotype threat.

Then, the men redid the walking test. This time Patrick walked faster than their usual walking speeds. While Naveen was still held back by the negative aging stereotype, the positive words had given Patrick a boost and reminded him of his true potential.

"Slower pace? Sounds like a nightmare!" says the aging athlete.

"Especially for one who is trying to qualify," I reply. Yet, stereotype threat can be a real issue for aging athletes, and it can be evoked so easily on race day, when you're asked your age and assigned to an age group to determine your start time. The underlying assumption is that the younger athletes will be faster than you, and from a purely biological standpoint, this is true. But our mind exaggerates the difference. I felt this at Mont Tremblant as I stood there watching those 20-somethings bound into the water at full speed, wishing I still had that much energy. That mere thought could have slowed me down.

Why Do Stereotypes Exist?

Our stereotypical brain creates a "quick-and-dirty" rule about people who belong to the same group, and then it automatically applies that rule whenever it encounters someone from that group. Unfortunately, as my daughter so aptly demonstrated, the "quick-and-dirty" rule for aging is **decline**. While it is true that decline *is* part of the aging process, not all of us will decline at the same rate. How far down will you decline? How fast? It depends on both your genes and your lifestyle.

You may have inherited an unhealthy set of genes that increases your risk of decline, but it doesn't guarantee your fate. The **apolipoprotein E (APOE)** gene has different versions, and its **ε4 allele** version increases your risk of dementia. One in four people inherit this unhealthy version, but it does not mean they will get dementia. Nor does it mean that people with the healthy version are protected. Why? Because lifestyle matters too, and it matters more than you may think.

Research from my lab has shown that **being physically inactive can**

completely negate a healthy set of genes.[6] Across 1,600 older adults, we found that those who were inactive had a similar risk of developing dementia as those who were genetically predisposed. This result suggests that your activity level contributes to your dementia risk as much as your genetics. **You can't change your genes, but you can change your lifestyle.**

To help explain this further, I'm going to put on my professor hat and give you a grade for your brain health. It will be similar to a grade you'd get on a report card, and just like in school, your grade will depend on a combination of two things:

1. Your natural ability (your genes)

2. Your work ethic (your habits)

My best students are not necessarily the smartest, but they definitely work the hardest. You may not be born with an A+ set of genes, but you can still get a passing grade in brain health by doing your work. Your homework? Exercise.

There are countless examples of exceptional people earning an A+ in aging. Kathrine Switzer, a Boston Marathon finisher who has overcome her fair share of discrimination in sports, is one. In 1967, during the Boston Marathon, officials humiliated her when they tried to rip off her bib midrace in an attempt to disqualify her. Why? Because she was a woman. Although there was no rule that prevented women from competing, the general opinion was that women were incapable — *too fragile, too weak, they might break, better not push it.* Switzer did not let their narrow-minded opinions stop her, and she became the first woman to officially register and complete the Boston Marathon (despite officials' attempts to stop her). Boston strong!

In 2017, Switzer, then 70 years old, ran the Boston Marathon again. Similar concerns circulated, but this time, not because of her gender but because of her age — *too fragile, too weak, she might break, better not push it.* Again, Switzer did not let their narrow-minded opinions stop her, and she completed the marathon in 4 hours and 44 minutes, just 24 minutes shy of her initial time 20 years prior. However, this time, Switzer was not alone. Over 200 seniors raced with her, including 33 women.

Eighty-four-year-old Katherine Beiers was among them, and the following year, at the ripe old age of 85, Beiers became the oldest woman to ever finish the Boston Marathon. Boston strong!

Master Athletes

Switzer and Beiers belong to a small but growing contingent of seniors who have earned the distinction of **master athlete**. How did they earn such distinction? By maintaining a high level of physical activity throughout their lives. But it's so much more than just a title; being a master athlete comes with tremendous health benefits too.

Fortunately, you don't have to run a marathon to earn an A+ in aging. I know so many incredible older people who deserve an honorary master's degree:

- Teng, who outrode me in a bike challenge last summer.
- Martin, who routinely outlifts me at our local gym.
- Sandy, who after a stroke was told she'd never walk again, gets out her cane and walks every day.

Want to become a master in aging?
Not sure where to start?
Start here!
I've prepared a short master's level course on brain health and aging to get you started.

AGING 101: A MASTER'S COURSE ON BRAIN HEALTH AND AGING

Please find enclosed a welcome message from your professor.

Dear Class,
Welcome to Aging 101; I'm excited to be your instructor. In this course, you will learn about the brain health benefits of being physically active. The course is broken down into **four** units. Each unit includes:

1. A set of required readings that examine the latest evidence.

2. An assignment where you will try out these evidence-based techniques on your own.

By the end of this course, you will have the knowledge and skill set to start your journey toward optimal brain health, regardless of your age or athletic ability.

Yours in good health,
Dr. Heisz

Unit 1: Take a Stand

Required Readings

1A) SITTING IS THE NEW SMOKING: A CASE STUDY

Here's the scenario: ~~You're busy at work.~~ Your *mind* is busy at work.

Your body just sits there. All day. Every day. With little to no movement.

You rush home. "Can we call that exercise?" you ask.

"Not unless you're walking or biking," I clarify.

You're not. In fact, you're sitting again. This time in traffic.

Finally, home. You're hungry and tired. You feed, TV, sleep, wake, and repeat.

It's the weekend. Tag! You're it. The kids run circles around you. You try to catch them but can't. You're *waaay* too out of breath. "When did I get so out of shape?" you wonder.

Time for your annual checkup. Not the clean bill of health you were hoping for. High blood pressure. Really? 130 over 80. "Is it serious?" you ask. Your doctor nods and advises: Less salt and alcohol. More fruits and vegetables. And try to get some exercise. You improve your diet but not your exercise habits. It helps a little but not a lot.

A year later, you're back at the doctor's office at risk for cardiovascular disease. Really? "We'll need to start monitoring you for heart disease, stroke, and dementia," your doctor explains.

"Getting *old* sucks!" you think.

But what you really mean to say is "Getting *unhealthy* sucks." And it does.

1B) FROM SITTING TO DEMENTIA IN THREE STEPS

"Wait, how did I go from high blood pressure to dementia?" you wonder.

"It's easier than you think," I explain. The health of your body has a direct impact on the health of your brain. In fact, there are only three degrees of separation between sitting too much and dementia.

1. You **sit** for long periods of time. Your body goes into hibernation mode, depressing your metabolism and increasing your **blood pressure**, blood sugar, and weight.[7]

2. Your high blood pressure damages your heart and its vessels. The small vessels that feed your brain get blocked, putting you at risk of **small vessel disease**. Without adequate blood supply, the brain's white matter starves to death.[8] White matter acts like a telephone wire that connects brain regions so they can talk to each other. When your white matter is damaged, the communication between those brain regions breaks down just like it did in that telephone game we played as kids; in the end, the message is all mixed up and everyone is confused. It was funny back then, but it's not funny now. The white matter damage shows up like bright lights on your brain scan called **white matter hyperintensities**. The scary part is that your brain could be lit up like a Christmas tree but clinically silent, meaning that you may have no noticeable symptoms until it's too late.[9]

3. Your extensive white matter damage causes faster **cognitive decline** and puts you at risk for dementia, stroke, and even death.[10] White matter hyperintensities are part of the main pathology for **vascular dementia**, the second leading cause of dementia. The blockage of the small vessels that feed the front regions of the brain impairs your executive functions more than your memory.[11] What about **Alzheimer's disease?** Reduced blood flow to the hippocampus puts you at risk for Alzheimer's

too.[12] However, the hippocampus has a back-up blood supply,[13] which means that its small vessels can tolerate more blockage before memory loss occurs. Vascular dementia and Alzheimer's often co-occur, and when they do, it's called **mixed dementia**.[14]

So, you see how easy it is to go from prolonged sitting to dementia. In fact, it's estimated that 30 percent of your dementia risk is tied to your sedentary lifestyle.[15] Sadly, some of the most sedentary people in the world are those with dementia.[16] For some patients, the most active part of their day is when their personal support worker transfers them from the bed to the chair and back again. Needless to say, their inactivity only serves to worsen their mental and physical health, hastening their decline. But it doesn't have to be *that* bad. And more to the point: All of this can be prevented. Your first assignment will help.

Your Assignment
Stand up!

"Right now?" you ask, confused.

"Yes, this is your assignment," I explain. Break up your sedentary time with short but frequent movement breaks using the protocol described below:

Every 30 minutes, stand up for a 2-minute movement break.

This is especially important if you are sitting for **4 or more hours**. Why? Sitting for that long reduces your brain's blood flow, and we just learned how bad this is for your brain's health. One study examined whether stand-up breaks could prevent the reduced blood flow from sitting continuously for 4 hours by testing three different protocols:[17]

1. Stand up for a 2-minute movement break every 30 minutes.

2. Stand up for an 8-minute movement break every 2 hours.

3. Sit continuously.

Although both break types included the same amount of stand-up time, the people who took shorter, more frequent breaks had more brain blood flow compared to the people who sat continuously.

Now over forty studies have examined the effect of breaking up sedentary time with short but frequent movement breaks,[18] and the general consensus is this: Breaking up prolonged sedentary time with short movement breaks prevents your body from going into hibernation mode. This reduces your likelihood of metabolic depression and your risk for high blood pressure, type 2 diabetes, and obesity, all of which reduce your risk for dementia.

Congratulations! You've completed your first assignment. Time to give yourself a standing ovation! Assignment grade = B+

Keep it up!

Unit 2: Interval Walking

Required Readings

2A) SIT VERSUS FIT: THE ULTIMATE MATCHUP

Although sitting may be as bad as smoking, some people can sit all day without any dire consequence. Who are those people? They are the most active among us. One study compiled data from over a million people.[19] At baseline, participants were asked about their daily activity habits regarding how much they:

1. Engaged in moderate to vigorous physical activity

2. Sat

3. Watched TV

Then, for up to 18 years, the researchers tracked death rates from all causes. Here's what they found: **Inactive people** had the highest death rate, and that rate increased the longer they sat and watched TV. The **most active people** had the lowest death rate. And those who walked briskly for at least an hour a day were able to **neutralize the detrimental effects of sitting for 8 hours and watching TV for 4 hours**.

The bottom line: If you like watching TV, then you'd better start moving.

2B) FITNESS REDUCES DEMENTIA RISK

What is it about being physically active that protects us from dementia? To help us answer this question, let's take a closer look at those master athletes. Their lifelong physical activity safeguards their bodies and minds against the deleterious effects of aging. Endurance athletes are not only **fitter** than their peers, they are just as fit as untrained young adults. Likewise, power athletes are not only **stronger** than their peers, they are just as strong as untrained young adults.[20]

Master athletes **live longer** too. One study tracked 900 male Olympians for about 52 years.[21] Their brothers were included as a control group to rule out genetic factors that impact longevity. The results were clear and highlighted the major role that lifestyle plays in determining our lifespan. Compared to their brothers, the Olympians maintained a high level of activity throughout their life that included **less sitting** and **more vigorous exercise**, and they lived longer because of it. However, some sports were more effective at extending lifespan than others. Although the power athletes enjoyed an additional 2 years of life over their brothers, the endurance athletes enjoyed an additional 7 *years*.

What is *so* good about endurance sports? Two words: **cardiorespiratory fitness**. When the heart (cardio) and lungs (respiratory) are functioning optimally, the rest of the body does too, including the brain. The gold standard for assessing your cardiorespiratory fitness is the **VO_2 max test**. Although the typical aging process is marred by a 12-percent-per-decade decline in VO_2 max, a master endurance athlete's fitness declines at half that rate, suggesting that at least half of our age-related loss of fitness is preventable with exercise.[22]

Regardless of whether you are a master athlete, having **higher fitness in midlife** protects you against developing dementia later in life. To demonstrate this link, one study recruited over 2,000 middle-aged men.[23] At baseline, the men performed a VO_2 max test and were grouped according to their relative fitness level. Then, over the next 22 years, the researchers tracked who developed dementia. Here's what they found:

- Dementia risk was nearly twice as high for the less fit than the more fit.
- Increasing VO_2 max by *3.5 ml/kg/min* reduced dementia risk by 20 percent.

And, yes, similar results have been observed for women.[24]

2C) STEPPING UP YOUR FITNESS

"How hard is it to increase my fitness by 3.5 points?" you ask, with fingers crossed that it's not too intensive. Today is your lucky day! Depending on your fitness level, walking may do the trick unless you're already a regular walker; in that case, you'll need to step it up. How? With intervals. When done in **midlife**, interval walking:

1. Increases your VO_2 max by about five points, especially if you're less fit.

2. Decreases your blood pressure, especially if it's high.

3. Improves your blood sugar regulation, especially if you have type 2 diabetes.

And interval walking does all of this better than regular walking.[25, 26, 27]

The best part? All three of these things lower your dementia risk too.

"When exactly *is* **midlife**?" you wonder, hoping it's not too late.

Some say midlife is between 40 and 60 years old.

Others extend that age range from 30 to 75.

"Seems ambitious!" you joke.

"Fingers crossed we all make it to 150 years old," I tease.

But all kidding aside, midlife is less about defining the middle point of your life and more about separating life's afternoon from its evening.[28] Defining midlife is more an art than a science. However, one thing is for sure: When midlife ends, old age starts. It's a time in our life when the sun is just starting to set. Just look at all that beauty on the horizon. It'd be a shame to miss it.

Your Assignment

Instead of going for your regular walk, try intermittently picking up the pace. Here is the standard interval walking protocol, i.e., the Wellness Walk Plus (page 115):

- Walk for 3 minutes at an easy pace.
- Walk for 3 minutes at a faster pace.
- Repeat five times.

You will know if you're walking fast enough when it becomes too difficult to talk.

Remember the **Talk Test**[29] from Chapter 1? You can use that test here to set your pace: Start exercising and ask yourself, "Can I talk comfortably right now?" If you answer yes, then this is a good pace for the easy intervals.

Pick up the pace and ask yourself again, "Can I talk comfortably right now?" When your answer is no, then it's a good pace for the faster intervals.

Bonus Assignment

How will you know when your fitness is improving? When you're able to cover more distance in the same amount of time. This is the basic principle of the **6-Minute Walk Test**, which you can do to determine your current fitness level. Researchers have developed a free app called the 6WT that uses GPS to track how far you walk.[30] All you need to do is set your age and sex, press play, and walk as far as you can in 6 minutes. Walk outdoors. Wear your normal walking shoes. Use a walking aid if you need to. Slow down or stop at any point. Do the test at least twice on 2 different days, preferably at the same time of day, and take the average of the 2.

My mom did the 6WT. Her average score was 0.4 mile. Way to go, Mom! Most people walk between 0.25 and 0.44 mile in 6 minutes. People who walk farther tend to have a higher VO_2 max[31] and therefore a lower risk of developing dementia.[32]

Congratulations! You've completed your second assignment. Assignment Grade = A-

You are learning fast!

Unit 3: Picking Up the Intensity

Required Readings

3A) THE IMPORTANCE OF BEING ABOVE YOUR LACTATE THRESHOLD

A walk a day keeps dementia at bay — that is, until you've increased your fitness so much that you can still talk comfortably at your fastest walking pace.

"Is that bad?" you ask, knowing full well that *that* is where you're at.

"No, it's great!" I explain. "It means your fitness has improved, and you're ready for the next step."

"Um, next step?" You hesitate. "To be completely honest, I'm *really* comfortable here."

That's the problem. You'll get more brain benefits with more challenging exercise. Not maximal effort but comfortably challenging, ideally at or slightly above your lactate threshold. Remember your "just-right" exercise intensity from Chapter 1? Right there!

Choose an activity you like; anything will do, so long as it is challenging enough: jogging . . . biking . . . swimming . . . dancing. You can use the Talk Test to know when you're ready to level up. Keep asking yourself, "Can I talk comfortably right now?" You need the answer to be no at least some of the time to give your brain the lactate it needs.

We talked about lactate in Chapter 1, but here's a quick refresher: Recall that lactate is produced when your working muscles need more fuel than oxygen can supply. To cover the shortfall, **anaerobic** metabolism kicks in, producing lactate. When lactate accumulates in the muscles, they become acidic and you feel the burn.

"Sounds toxic!" you exclaim, and for a long time, scientists thought the same. However, it turns out that lactate is not toxic at all, especially for the brain. Ironically, lactate helps protect the brain against the toxic effects of dementia in *two* important ways:

1. Lactate enhances blood flow to the brain by building new blood vessels.

   - During midlife, the blood flow to the brain decreases at a rate of about 10 percent per decade.[33] Lactate, which builds up during vigorous exercise, stimulates the production of more blood vessels in the brain to increase blood flow.[34] Therefore, exercising above your lactate threshold gives your brain the lactate it needs to ward off **vascular dementia**.

2. Lactate fuels neuroplasticity by promoting the growth and function of brain cells.

   - Lactate travels from the exercising muscles to the hippocampus, where it increases **brain-derived neurotrophic factor (BDNF)**.[35] BDNF acts like a fertilizer for brain cells, helping them grow, but it is reduced in the hippocampus of individuals with Alzheimer's.[36] Therefore, exercising above your lactate threshold gives your brain the lactate it needs to ward off **Alzheimer's**.

3B) A (VERY) BRIEF HISTORY OF NEUROGENESIS

For a long time, scientists believed that, after a critical period in early childhood, the brain's wiring was fixed for life. "Adding or removing brain cells would ruin the brain's intricate neural circuitry and disrupt the flow of neural communication to cause dysfunction," said one archaic professor to another, and both men nodded their heads in agreement. This misbelief was so ingrained that initial evidence to the contrary[37] was highly criticized and outright rejected. "These researchers must be wrong," said those same men to their archaic professor friends, and all the men nodded their heads in agreement.

That was until 1999, when a bright young woman named Henriette van Praag published a series of studies that began to convince the scientific community otherwise,[38, 39] and her research fundamentally changed the way we viewed the aging brain. A key discovery was that **neurogenesis** (the birth of new brain cells) could occur in adulthood — but it only occurred in certain regions. The primary site? The hippocampus.

Another key discovery was that the most effective way to grow new brain cells was by exercising. Exercising induced neurogenesis[40] and improved memory[41] in young mice and **old** mice too.[42] In fact, it was almost as if exercising had made the old brains young again.

3C) DO HUMAN BRAINS GROW NEW BRAIN CELLS TOO?

This is the million-dollar question and one that is still hotly debated. Just a few years ago, a month apart, two high-profile studies were published. One found evidence of human neurogenesis[43] whereas the other did not.[44] Although most scientists believe human neurogenesis exists, the challenge is that we can't measure neurogenesis in live humans. Instead, we have to wait until after death to directly examine the brain, and there tend to be vast inconsistencies in the time between death and examination that can alter the results. As a workaround, researchers rely on *two* indirect measures that can be done while the person is still alive and well:

1. **Sizing up the hippocampus.** A common proxy for neurogenesis is to measure the size of the hippocampus using MRI.

   - With advancing age, the hippocampus shrinks at a rate of 1.5 percent per year in healthy older adults and 4 percent per year in Alzheimer's patients.[45]
   - Exercise counteracts the expected decline and may even reverse it. Older adults who walked three times per week for a year enjoyed a 2 percent increase in their hippocampal volume.[46]
   - After just 3 months of walking/jogging, older adults whose fitness improved also experienced greater increases in their hippocampal size and blood flow.[47]
   - However, one problem with sizing up the hippocampus this way is that MRI cannot distinguish new brain cells from other cells; nevertheless, this method still clearly demonstrates a significant effect of exercise on the brains of older adults.

2. **Testing hippocampal function.** Newborn neurons fit together like the pieces of a puzzle. Each puzzle piece represents a different aspect of a memory. When you have more puzzle pieces, then you can create richer memories that are less fallible to error.

   There are different forms of memory and not all of them depend on the hippocampus. Because of this, some aspects of memory are more or less affected by aging, Alzheimer's, and exercise.

   > **Episodic memory** refers to our memory for events. It is most dependent on the hippocampus and declines with aging[48] and Alzheimer's disease.[49] This is why a person with Alzheimer's finds it hard to recognize familiar faces, remember whether she took her medication today or yesterday, or locate her parked car in a busy parking lot.

   > **Procedural memory** refers to our memory for skills and actions. It is less dependent on the hippocampus. This is why a person in the early stages of Alzheimer's can still remember how to ride a bike.

Semantic memory refers to our memory for facts. It is less dependent on the hippocampus. This is why a person in the early stages of Alzheimer's disease can still remember the lyrics to her favorite childhood song.

My lab tested out the effect of interval walking on episodic memory.[50] Sixty-four sedentary but cognitively healthy seniors enrolled in our community-based program held at our local seniors' gym called the Physical Activity Centre of Excellence (PACE). Exercise sessions were supervised, three times a week for 12 weeks, using the following protocol:

- Light walking for 3 minutes.
- Vigorous walking for 4 minutes.
- Repeat four times.

As the participants' fitness improved, we increased the speed or incline of the treadmill to achieve the target intensity.

After just 12 weeks of interval walking, the seniors' episodic memory had improved by 30 percent, and their improvement in memory was directly related to their fitness gains. What's more, memory only improved for the seniors who interval walked. Memory did not improve for the seniors who walked regularly or stretched.

Taken together, the results suggest that high-intensity interval exercise (that is challenging enough to increase lactate above its threshold) may be an ideal type of exercise to improve memory and keep dementia at bay.

Your Assignment

When interval walking becomes too easy for you, try one of these high-intensity interval training (HIIT) protocols:

Interval walking up and down a hill. Check out the Memory Booster on page 116.

Interval walking on a treadmill. Play with the pace and incline.

Interval biking by increasing your resistance and cadence.

Interval swimming by picking up the pace.

HIIT it for your brain health! Grade = A
Excellent effort!

Unit 4: Group Work

Required Readings

4A) THE EXERCISE PILL

Alzheimer's disease clutters the brain with amyloid plaques and tau tangles, which kill brain cells and impair cognition. Unfortunately, there have been several failed attempts at finding a cure — first with drugs that targeted amyloid and then with drugs that targeted tau. But hope has been renewed with the discovery of a new hormone called **irisin**.[51]

The latest breakthrough? Alzheimer's brains are irisin-deficit.[52] Exercising helps correct that deficit, but what's more, these exercise effects are mimicked by simply injecting irisin into the bloodstream to improve memory and reduce the severity of Alzheimer's disease. Although this initial research was done in animals, the latest research suggests that it may work the same way in humans too.[53, 54] One can only hope this new research will lead to a cure for Alzheimer's. It may even lead to the creation of the elusive exercise pill, which would be transformative for patients in the severe stages of Alzheimer's who are unable to exercise.

On second thought, wouldn't it be nice if we could *all* take an exercise pill? I'll admit, it sounded appealing, especially on our drive to Lake Placid. The time had come for my half Ironman world championship qualifying race. I had recruited one of my new exercise friends to do it with me, and we were both anticipating at least a 5-hour grueling battle. By the end of it all, our brains would be bathed in lactate, BDNF, and irisin! Could an exercise pill do the same?

The idea of an exercise pill is likely too good to be true. Why? Because not all of exercise's benefits can be reduced to a single molecule and bottled up. Can you fit all your exercise friends into a bottle? Absolutely not! And this is the real reason an exercise pill will never be able to replace the real deal.

4B) LIFELONG EXERCISE

Exercise friends are also one of the main reasons people stay motivated to exercise their entire life. Meet Mark. He's a master runner who has been running for more than 8 years. What got him started and what keeps him coming back after all these years? "I came for the physical. Stayed for the psychological. And remained steadfastly motivated for the social," he said. And all of Mark's running friends agreed.[55]

But perhaps the strongest support for the social benefits of exercise can be seen in people with **mild cognitive impairment (MCI)**, character-ized by a slight but noticeable decline in memory that is often associated with poor physical health.[56] When it comes to brain health, MCI is a kind of no-man's land. People with MCI don't have dementia, but they're not healthy either. Some stay there. Some progress to dementia. Others revert to normal, especially if their problems with high blood pressure are addressed.[57]

"Revert to normal?" you ask in bewilderment.

"Yes, back to normal," I confirm, and exercising increases those odds. One study found that **24 percent of people with MCI scored "normal"** after just 6 months of supervised resistance training — a reversion rate that was three times higher than that of a control group.[58]

Yet, despite these incredible brain health benefits, many people with MCI quit exercising after the supervised part of the study was over. Although 85 percent of participants with MCI are able to complete a supervised group-based exercise program, only 25 percent are able to continue being physically active on their own.[59] It raises the question: Why aren't supervised group-based exercise programs for MCI running continuously?

4C) THE SOCIAL BRAIN

To our social brain, one *is* the loneliest number, and there are two ways it can be *one:*

1. You may be **socially isolated** because you don't have enough people around.

2. You may be **lonely** because you *feel* alienated.

You can be socially isolated without feeling lonely and feel lonely without being socially isolated. In all cases, your brain lacks the social stimulation it needs, and because of this, it withers and your faculties fade. Being either socially isolated or feeling lonely increases your risk of developing dementia.[60, 61]

To help socially isolated seniors, the solution may be as simple as providing more opportunities for them to socialize. I personally think every neighborhood should have a senior walk/run club or a seniors' gym like PACE.

- Seniors prefer exercising with their peers, who, and I quote, "understand the aches and pains of the older persons."[62]
- The exercise program should be close to home, affordable, and easy to access.
- And most importantly, it should be *fun*, with lots of opportunity to laugh and form friendships.

Seniors who have an "exercise family" are more social, feel more supported, and are more likely to adhere to an exercise program over the long term,[63] which does a brain good.

It does a body good too. Seniors who exercise regularly with others report being healthier than those who exercise alone, and this is true regardless of how much they actually exercise.[64] Most importantly, seniors who exercise together feel less *lonely*,[65] which helps prevent this more challenging situation to solve.

Here's the scenario: Lawrence is a lonely senior. He became lonely soon after his wife died. The challenge with Lawrence's loneliness is that it makes him feel **unsafe**.[66]

His lonely brain is hypervigilant. When it's faced with the choice of fight or flight, it wants to *flee* far away from the world and everyone in it. The worst part? Through a lonely lens, Lawrence sees a lonely world. He expects social interactions to be negative, and because of his bias, he experiences all social interactions that way. Unfortunately for Lawrence, his loneliness has become a self-fulfilling prophecy where he pushes people away to feel "safe" only to alienate himself further.

It goes without saying that lonely people like Lawrence are less likely to be physically active, and if they happen to be active now, they are less likely to stay active over time.[67]

Fortunately, Lawrence is not lonely anymore. **Supervised exercise**

helped to reduce his loneliness. It was the baby step that he needed to renew his trust in the world. It helped that his trainer used a compassionate approach. Rather than focusing solely on strengthening Lawrence's body, his trainer designed a fun, achievable, and social program that was focused on:[68]

- Alleviating his concerns about safety.
- Overcoming his self-limiting biases.
- Helping him gain confidence in his abilities.

Thanks to his supervised exercise program, Lawrence enjoys life again. He's stronger, healthier, more confident, more independent, and more engaged. He's even started exercising on his own. In fact, his daily walk around the park with his dear friend is one of the highlights of his day.

4D) A HEALTHY BRAIN MAKES IT EASIER TO EXERCISE

We have one final topic to cover before we end the course (and the chapter). Up to this point, I've focused your curriculum on the benefits of exercise for brain health. However, it is important to acknowledge that the opposite is true too. One's ability to engage in exercise depends on having a healthy brain, which means it's harder to exercise when you're cognitively impaired. Unfortunately, this is why many people with dementia spend most of their day sedentary. But it doesn't have to be that way.

Meet Betty, an 85-year-old woman with dementia. Her condition is mild, which means she still has full control over her body, though it's not safe for her to exercise on her own because her risk of falling is too high.[69] So, Betty just sits there all day every day—that is, until her favorite nephew buys her a brand-new stationary bike (recumbent, not racer) and hooks it up to her TV. Betty—carefully, with assistance—hops on her new bike and goes for a virtual ride through the familiar streets of her hometown. "Ahh, it brings back such great memories," Betty reminisces, using all of her semantic memory that is still intact. Her sweetheart nephew knows she likes Sinatra and cranks the tunes. And there's Betty on her new bike, bombing around in her hometown, singing at the top of her lungs. Tears fill her nephew's eyes. He hasn't seen her this alive in years. Her brain is prospering; her body is too.[70] Sure beats just sitting there watching TV.

But let's do Betty one better. Let's give her a multiplayer online cycling community so she can interact, train, and compete with other seniors in a virtual world. Instead of biking aimlessly, Betty's now out on a biking adventure with her friends. She's laughing out loud, joking around with her dear friends like she's back in high school. They race each other on their recumbents through the streets of their hometown. Betty wins! "Hooray!" the crowd cheers. Betty's avatar jumps up on the podium (unassisted) to claim her gold medal. Betty smiles, and her avatar takes a bow.

"Hip-hip-hooray! Three cheers for Betty," the crowd cheers. Hip-hip-hooray for Betty and her better quality of life!

Your Assignment
Make one of your weekly workouts a group activity.

Your group can be two or more. Virtual groups count too. You may want to choose to do something other than walking. Check out the Vitality Pump or the Elixir for Life workouts on pages 115 and 116. According to a recent review that compiled the result of thirty-six exercise interventions, your options are endless.[71] For people over 50 years old, living in the community (without dementia but possibly with cognitive impairment), the following exercises have been shown to improve cognition:

Type	Aerobic Strength Multicomponent (aerobic plus resistance) Tai chi
Intensity	At least moderate
Duration	45 to 60 minutes
Frequency	On as many days as feasible
Length	At least 4 weeks

Grade = A+
Time for your gold medal finish!

"Speaking of gold medal," one reader interjects, "how did *your* race go?"

"It was no walk in the park," I admit, "but I gave it my all and finished fifth in my age group, which was fast enough to earn a qualifying spot for the world championships."

"Hip-hip-hooray!" you cheer.

"They even let me jump up on the podium," I laugh, still in disbelief. But then my tone quiets. "To be completely honest, my victory was bittersweet because my friend didn't qualify. I really wish she had. It would have been better together."

And on that note, you call up a friend, lace up your running shoes, and head to the park. Once around, maybe twice, picking up the pace intermittently, of course. Smiling and laughing too. "Shall we go for three?" you ask your friend with fingers crossed, not wanting the fun to end. "Hip-hip-hooray!" your friend cheers, and you both keep walking.

The Extender Workout

REFERENCE: Chapter 5
MINDSET: Fit for life

NEURO FIX: Nourish the brain with vital nutrients
LEVEL: Intermediate

MON	TUES	WED	THURS	FRI	SAT	SUN
Wellness Walk	Vitality Pump	Wellness Walk Plus		Memory Booster	Elixir for Life	

WELLNESS WALK

Walk for 30 minutes at a comfortable, easy pace. Pay attention to your breathing.

VITALITY PUMP

Warm up with a 5-minute Wellness Walk, then complete exercises 1 to 6 for the prescribed repetitions. Take a 30-second mindful break. Focus on your breathing. Repeat.

ORDER	EXERCISE	REPETITIONS	PICTURED
1	Kickouts	10 reps per side	Page 178
2	Supine Hip Lifts	10 reps	Page 198
3	Superman (alternating)	10 reps per side	Page 197
4	Sit Stands	10 reps	Page 192
5	Pushups (modified, wall)	10 reps	Page 185
6	Single-Leg Balance	10 reps per side	Page 191
	Mindful Break	30 seconds	

Ready to take the next step? Increase your repetitions to 15 reps and 40 seconds. Repeat the exercises a third time. *Advanced progressions:* 3. Superman (alternating) to Superman, hold each repetition for 5 seconds; 5. Pushups (modified, wall) to Pushups (modified); 6. Single Leg Balance to Single Leg Balance with eyes closed.

WELLNESS WALK PLUS

Warm up with a 5-minute Wellness Walk, then pick up the pace until you can no longer talk comfortably (brisk walk or easy jog). Maintain that pace for 3 minutes. Then take a 3-minute Wellness Walk break. Alternate between faster and slower paces five times. Cool down with a 5-minute Wellness Walk.

Ready to take the next step? Add an extra repeat each week. Swap your regular Wellness Walk for a Wellness Walk Plus. Add more days.

MEMORY BOOSTER

Warm up with a 5-minute Wellness Walk. Walk up a gradual hill for 4 minutes and then walk down the hill. Repeat hill walk four times. Cool down with a 5-minute Wellness Walk.

Ready to take the next step? Add an extra repeat each week. Try a steeper hill.

ELIXIR FOR LIFE

Warm up with a 5-minute Wellness Walk, then complete exercises 1 to 6 for the prescribed repetitions. Take a 30-second mindful break. Focus on your breathing. Repeat.

ORDER	EXERCISE	REPETITIONS	PICTURED
1	Front Plank (modified)	30 seconds	Page 175
2	Bird Dogs	10 reps per side	Page 169
3	Squats (supported)	10 reps	Page 195
4	Side-Lying Hip Abduction	10 reps per side	Page 189
5	Lateral Raises (bent over)	10 reps	Page 182
6	Cat Cow	10 reps per movement	Page 171
	Mindful Break	30 seconds	

Ready to take the next step? Increase your repetitions to 15 reps and 40 seconds. Repeat the exercises a third time. *Advanced progressions:* 1. Front Plank (modified) to Front Plank; 3. Squats (supported) to Squats.

$$6$$

MOVE MORE TO SLEEP, THINK, AND FEEL BETTER

Go to bed; you'll feel better in the morning.

— MY MOM

YOU WORK HARD juggling all of your priorities and striving for that elusive work–life balance. Is it actually achievable? I'm not sure. Your to-do list seems longer than life itself. Where's your workout on that list? At the bottom.

At times, you are so busy that you don't even sleep, but you pay for it the next day.

Too tired to think.

Too sleepy to smile.

Too exhausted to exercise.

You need your sleep, and for some reason this lesson is hard to learn.

One night of insufficient sleep becomes two. Then four. Then ten. Weeks go by. Months even. You grow weary with fatigue, and the consequences escalate. You're making major mistakes at work. Feeling depressed and anxious. And, to top it all off, you're gaining weight.

When you finally have enough time to sleep, it's hard to fall asleep and stay asleep.

How many times did you get up last night? Too many to count.

You try to self-medicate with alcohol, but it makes you feel worse.

A coffee a day keeps your sleepiness at bay but only temporarily.

Your doctor recommends exercise, and you reluctantly agree.

"Didn't you just say I was too exhausted to exercise?" you ask.

I did.

But some is better than none, and the more you move, the better you sleep.

Now you're moving more and sleeping better, thinking better, and feeling better too.

And you're not too tired to exercise. "Same time tomorrow?" you ask because you know that consistent exercise helps you fall asleep faster.

"One more hill repeat?" you insist because you know that intense exercise helps you sleep more soundly.

In this chapter, I'll first describe how sleeplessness affects your ability to think, feel, and exercise. Then, I'll explain how you can use exercise to reset your brain so you fall asleep faster and sleep more soundly.

ARE YOU SLEEPING ENOUGH?

About one in three people aren't sleeping enough, including me, and this is making it harder to be healthy. The number one sleep complaint? **Insomnia**, which includes difficulty falling asleep and staying asleep. Although insomnia — the disorder — only affects about 10 percent of the population, 30 percent of us will experience insomnia *symptoms* from time to time, and that prevalence is higher among women, older adults, and people with mental illness.[1]

I am all too familiar with the pains of insomnia, the symptoms of which have been part and parcel of my OCD for years.[2] My symptoms were never bad enough to amount to a clinical disorder — that is, they never persisted for 3 or more nights a week and for longer than 3 months.[3] However, I would argue that that's a pretty steep criteria, especially given that I could feel the shortfall from a single night of disrupted sleep.

Since I started this fitness journey, I'm happy to report that my sleep has improved tremendously. Is it perfect? No, at least not every night. But one thing is certain: When I exercise during the day, I sleep better at night. In fact, over the course of the last 2½ years, I've come to really appreciate the benefits of exercise for sleep — so much so that I now consider sleep to be one of the greatest gifts that exercise gives. Why? Because it has the power to affect everything the brain does. And I do mean everything.

How Much Sleep Do You Actually Need and Why?

Sleep is vital for brain health, and without it, the brain doesn't function very well. The amount of sleep we need depends on our age. Kids and teens need more sleep than adults because their young brains and bodies are working hard to grow and develop. The National Sleep Foundation recommends the following:[4]

- Kids, 6 to 13 years old, should get 9 to 11 hours of sleep every night.
- Teens, 14 to 17 years old, should get 8 to 10 hours.
- Adults, 18 to 64 years old, should get 7 to 9 hours.
- Seniors, 65 years old and older, should get 7 to 8 hours.

Lazed in a comfy bed with head nestled on a soft pillow and body snuggled under a warm blanket. Doesn't that sound divine? Yet the business of our modern life has no time for sleep, not just for us adults but for kids and teens too. Consider a day in the life of one teen named Simon. On weekends, Simon stays up past midnight and sleeps until noon. Come Monday, he needs to be up and dressed by 7 a.m. for school. After school, it's extracurriculars, then homework, then social. It's already midnight.

"Go to bed!" Mom yells.

"I'm not tired!" Simon replies, without even looking up from his phone. The whole week is like this. Simon is supposed to be getting 8 to 10 hours of sleep a night. Although he might be getting that much on the weekends, he's definitely not getting that much on weekdays.

Unfortunately, Simon's schedule is the norm.[5] Sleep-deprived teenagers are taking over the world! What's even worse? The sleep habits we form as teens lay the foundation for how we will sleep as adults.[6]

Perhaps not surprisingly, a teenager holds the record for the longest amount of time a human has ever gone without sleep. In the 1960s, Randy Gardner took up the challenge for his high school science fair project. By the end of his 11-day experiment, Randy's brain had practically turned to mush. He couldn't remember things. It was as if he had Alzheimer's brought on by lack of sleep. But you don't have to be completely deprived to become senseless with sleeplessness. One bad night of sleep will do. And those short sleeps throughout the week (that we are all guilty of) really do add up.[7]

HOW SLEEP AFFECTS YOUR LIFE

Too Sleepy to Smile: How Sleep Affects Your Mood

As I alluded to before, sleeplessness is both a cause and a consequence of mental illness. People with mental illness are more likely to suffer from insomnia, and people with insomnia are nearly ten times more likely to be **depressed** and more than seventeen times more likely to be **anxious**.[8] Sleep deprivation impairs communication between the amygdala and prefrontal cortex (PFC).[9] Two things happen: anxiety and moodiness. Although we are all at risk, teens are especially vulnerable because the connection between their amygdala and PFC is still forming and may be more easily disrupted by poor sleep.[10]

To demonstrate the impact of sleeplessness on mood, one study recruited fifty teens. Simon was one of them.[11] When Simon's sleep was restricted to 6.5 hours per night (a typical schedule for him on the weekdays), he felt tired and had less vigor. He was also more **anxious**, **angry**, and **confused**. Simon's mom noted that he seemed more oppositional and moodier. Yet, she *failed to notice any significant change in his anxiety*, and herein lies a major point of concern. If we don't see our teen's anxiety, we can't help them, and they will continue to suffer alone. Most tragically, teens who have trouble sleeping in early adolescence are more likely to deliberately harm themselves or attempt suicide in late adolescence.[12]

I beg you, please, please, please ask your teens how they are sleeping. They may feel more comfortable talking to you about their poor sleep than their poor mental health, and it could be the conversation that saves a life. According to the U.S. Centers for Disease Control and Prevention, suicide is one of the leading causes of death for this age group, taking more lives per year than homicide and heart disease combined.[13] It doesn't have to be that way. If you or someone you know is not sleeping well, there may be a bigger mental health issue at hand. Seek help when you need it. Call the National Suicide Prevention Lifeline at 1-800-273-TALK (8255), or text the Crisis Text Line (text HELLO to 741741).

Too Tired to Think: Microsleep When You Least Expect It

Less tragic but still not ideal, a poor night's sleep can also make us look dumb. Here's the scenario: You're in the middle of a meeting. The boss is up front giving instructions, but you're tired and stare at her blankly. Suddenly, your head drops. You jerk awake. Eyes refocus. You see your boss. Why is she staring at you? Did she ask you a question? "Um, five hundred?" you reply. Wrong. In fact, *so* wrong. Unfortunately, she's not asking you about finances. Doh! "Can anyone else answer the question?" your boss begs, now annoyed. Almost everyone raises their hand. She picks the woman beside you. "It's October 10, 2019, World Mental Health Day," she answers before looking your way and smiling smugly. She obviously slept much better than you did last night.

Of course, you could have correctly answered that question too. The problem was that you didn't hear it. You didn't hear it because your brain was sleeping. Not a regular close-your-eyes-for-8-hours kind of sleep, but a **microsleep** that lasts mere moments.[14] Microsleeps happen during the day when the brain doesn't get enough sleep at night. It takes your consciousness offline for a few seconds to restore function.[15] Just a few seconds, what's the harm in that? Unfortunately, a lot of things can happen in just a few seconds, sometimes very important things.

One study demonstrated the impact of sleeplessness on vigilance.[16] Sheryl was one of the participants. For 1 week, Sheryl's sleep was restricted to 5 hours a night, and her vigilance was tested every day. When rested, Sheryl only made two errors on the test. However, after just 1 night of restricted sleep, she made **four** errors. After 2 nights, **six**. After 4 nights, **twelve**. And after 1 week, **eighteen**. What's worse? Even after 2 good nights of sleep, Sheryl was still missing things because her vigilance had yet to fully recover.

Driving While Drowsy

Sleep restriction impairs driving too. Let me ask you a question: **Would you ever drive drunk?** The answer should be a resounding NO! We know that alcohol severely impairs our driving ability. Two to four drinks can increase your blood alcohol level above 0.05 percent, which severely impairs your ability to drive, and a blood alcohol level above 0.05 percent in Utah and 0.08 percent in all other states makes you legally unfit to drive. This is a criminal offense that can lead to jail time.

Let me ask you another question: **Would you ever drive drowsy?** In a national survey, one in five people admitted to driving drowsy in the last month, and 40 percent admitted to falling asleep at the wheel in the past year.[17] Eek! One study compared the effects of intoxication versus sleep deprivation on vigilance.[18] After 17 hours without sleep, the participants' vigilance was as bad as if they had a blood alcohol level of 0.05 percent. In other words, too intoxicated to drive.

Seventeen hours is really not that long. Truck drivers drive that tired all the time. Drowsy driving was the cause of the tragic accident that involved a truck driver who collided with a limo that left the actor Tracy Morgan with a head injury and killed his friend. The driver had been up for more than 24 hours straight. What was most shocking was that the driver didn't even slow down before the crash. It was as if he didn't see the limo. That's because he *didn't* see the limo. He was micro-sleeping.

Health care workers also work long hours. Medical interns routinely work shifts that last over 24 hours. One study compared the number of errors made during an extended 29-hour shift versus two shorter shifts of 15 and 14 hours.[19] During the extended shift, interns made 36 percent more serious medical errors and nearly six times more serious diagnostic errors than they did during the two shorter shifts. Would you want a drowsy surgeon operating on you? I don't think so.

Too Exhausted to Exercise (But Not to Eat)

If you're too tired to think, it's probably safe to assume you're too tired to exercise. In fact, restricting sleep for just 1 week makes people more sedentary.[20] Rosanna, a regular exerciser, and Sarah, who was already pretty sedentary, took part in a study that restricted their sleep to 5½ hours a night for 1 week. During that week, Rosanna reallocated about a third of her moderate to vigorous activity to light or sedentary activities, and Sarah became even more sedentary.

"Can't I sit here a little longer and eat cake?" asked Sarah before doing just that. You can probably see where this is going. The problem with insufficient sleep is that it doesn't just make you less active, it makes you eat more too.[21] Why? Two reasons:

1. When we sleep less, we are awake more. There is simply **more opportunity to eat**.
2. Also, a tired person eats more because their hormones are out of whack.
   - **Ghrelin** increases, which stimulates appetite.
   - **Leptin** decreases, which is needed to suppress appetite.

Moving less and eating more is the formula for weight gain. The pounds add up quickly and increase your risk of obesity.[22] We need to get ahead of our sleep problems before they get to that point.

The solution? We need to move more to sleep better, and once we are sleeping better, it will be easier for us to move more. It's a virtuous cycle!

When it comes to exercising for better sleep, the options are endless: walking, running, biking, strength training, yoga, and tai chi.[23, 24, 25] Some is better than none, but the more you move, the better you will sleep.[26] To top it off, there are even ways to optimize exercise to help you fall asleep faster and sleep more soundly. We will cover those next.

HOW EXERCISE AFFECTS YOUR SLEEP

Exercise and Getting to Sleep

Meet Irene. Irene has insomnia. In spite of having enough time to sleep, Irene struggles to fall asleep almost every night. Her brain time is way out of sync with real time. Fortunately, exercise can help reset Irene's brain time to help her fall asleep faster. Here's how it works.

Tick-tock goes our biological clock. Its rhythm is circadian. What time is it? Don't check your watch. It may be wrong. Why? Because our biological clock operates on its own time. Brain time is set by the **clock genes** in the **suprachiasmatic nucleus** of the brain. The body's schedule is programmed around brain time. Tomorrow's agenda is jam-packed with back-to-back meetings about protein production. What to make? How much to make? When to make it? Here's the agenda:

. . .

7 a.m.   Make morning proteins to wake up.

. . .

12 p.m.   Make afternoon proteins to digest lunch.

. . .

4 p.m.   Make midafternoon proteins to exercise.

. . .

11 p.m.   Make evening proteins to sleep.

. . .

Clock genes keep us on brain time. But there's one problem. Our clock genes run late, with an inherent tardiness that is built into our DNA. How late? Put it this way: in real time it takes **24 hours** for Earth to rotate on its axis, whereas in brain time a day is **24.2 hours**.[27] What's the extra **0.2 hour** (12 minutes) for? No one knows. But if left unchecked, brain time will tick completely out of sync with reality.

Let's say you were to live in a dark, secluded bunker with no natural light, clocks, or other clues about time (I know it sounds creepy, but stay with me). After 60 days, because your brain time has longer days, your sleep-wake cycle would be 100 percent opposite to what it is now. How do we know this? Scientists have actually tested it. Back in the 1960s, Dr. Jürgen Aschoff, the director of the Max Planck Institute in Germany, built a bunker and acted as his own guinea pig,[28] documenting how much his sleep-wake schedule changed from lack of light. While he lived in that dark bunker, Dr. Aschoff's brain time steadily shifted out of sync with clock time, and he fell asleep and woke up later and later every day.[29]

Resetting Brain Time with Melatonin and Exercise

Fortunately, we can turn back the hands of brain time to resync with real time. In fact, we do this every morning when the sun hits our eyes. Sunlight increases **melatonin** — one of nature's strongest sleeping aids.[30]

In the absence of modern-day electronic devices, melatonin rises and falls opposite to the sun. Unfortunately, the bright light from using tech at night can cause a **daylight savings–like shift** in melatonin, delaying its production and making it harder for us to fall asleep.[31] The brain also needs serotonin to make melatonin, which is why many people with **depression** sleep terribly and feel worse because of it.[32]

The solution? Put down your electronic device; put on your running shoes. It turns out that exercise can reset brain time too. One study determined the extent to which exercise and sunlight reset brain time and whether combining the two was better than using just one.[33] The study involved three separate lab visits. Steve was one of the participants, and on each visit, Steve slept for 1 hour (no light, in bed) then stayed awake for 2 hours (dim light, out of bed), and repeated this ultrashort sleep-wake schedule for 2.5 days straight. Why did they make him do that? So that his brain would completely lose track of time. Then, Steve completed one of three conditions: bright lights only, exercise only, or bright lights plus exercise.

During Steve's first visit, the **bright lights** were turned on at hour 30 for 90 minutes. The illumination intensity was 5,000 lux, which is ten times brighter than most offices. That was enough to delay Steve's brain time by **nearly 1 hour**.

During Steve's second visit, he **exercised** at hour 30 for 90 minutes. This was enough to delay Steve's brain time by **nearly 50 minutes**, almost as much as the bright lights.

During Steve's third and final visit, the **bright lights** were turned on at hour 30 for 90 minutes and he **exercised** at hour 36 for 90 minutes. The bright lights plus exercise delayed Steve's brain time by **1 hour and 20 minutes** for a synergistic effect!

How can you apply these lab results to real life? Exercise outside at the *same time every day*. Some is better than none, but **consistency** is key. Make the timing of your workouts as reliable as the sun. This will help keep your brain time aligned with real time so you can fall asleep faster.

Exercise Right for your Chronotype

You can personalize the timing of your workouts to match your own unique biological clock needs. Depending on your genes and lifestyle, you may want to synchronize your brain time to a slightly different schedule than me. This is your chronotype. You can exercise right for your chronotype. Here's how:

First, let's determine your chronotype. Imagine you have nothing to do tomorrow. Ask yourself the following questions:

1. What time will you go to sleep tonight?

2. What time will you wake up tomorrow?

Your preference reveals your chronotype. **Morning types** prefer to wake up really early. **Evening types** prefer to stay up really late. **Intermediate types** fall somewhere in between. I am undeniably an evening type. I'm not even going to tell you what time it is right now. It's *really* late. According to a recent survey of over 50,000 Americans, most people are intermediate types.[34] The study included men and women who were 15 years old and older.

25 percent are morning types.

50 percent are intermediate types.

25 percent are evening types.

The **sexes** differed in chronotype. Before 40 years old, men tended to stay up later than women. After 40, men tended to go to bed earlier than women.

Some **age groups** were dominated by certain chronotypes. Seniors had more morning types than any other age group. Teenagers had more evening types than any other age group. And herein lies the problem for teens. Their evening chronotype clashes with their early school start time. The average senior high school student prefers to go to bed around 1 a.m. This bedtime is okay on the weekends when they can sleep in, but it's not okay on the weekdays when they need to be up much earlier. What's worse? This sleep schedule causes **social jet lag** — their weekend-to-weekday transition is like traveling between two different time zones. From the East Coast to the West Coast and back again every week. How exhausting!

Social jet lag, **real jet lag, shift work** . . . any schedule that takes you out of sync with the sun is enough to confuse the brain and alter the release of melatonin, making it harder for you to fall asleep.

The solution? Try exercising at the same time every day. What time? Well, that depends on your chronotype.

HOW TO PERSONALIZE YOUR EXERCISE ALARM CLOCK

The same researchers who conducted the bright lights and exercise study conducted another ultrashort sleep schedule study.[35] As before, they scheduled sleep so the brain would lose track of time. However, in this study, participants slept on an ultrashort schedule for 3 days straight. Each day, the participants walked briskly on a treadmill for 60 minutes at a prespecified time (same time every day): 1 a.m., 4 a.m., 7 a.m., 10 a.m., 1 p.m., 4 p.m., 7 p.m., or 10 p.m.

"Who would participate in such a study?" you wonder. You are not going to believe this, but it's true. First of all, the researchers managed to recruit 101 people for this study. What's more, about half of them were young adults, while the other half were older adults between 59 and 75 years old. Seventy-five years old!

But regardless of the participant's age, the exercise induced daylight savings–like time shifts. Here's what they found:

- To get your brain time to "*fall back*," exercise in the morning at 7 a.m. and in the afternoon between 1 and 4 p.m.
- To get your brain time to "*spring forward*," exercise in the evening between 7 and 10 p.m.

Translation: If you're an evening type who wants to go to bed earlier, try exercising in the morning or afternoon. If you're a morning type who wants to stay up later, try exercising in the evening. It worked for a high school run club that got teens out of bed to exercise at 7 a.m. Not only did they fall asleep faster, but they also slept, thought, and felt better too.[36]

Advice on Exercise Before Bed

Listen up, morning types! I know what you're thinking: "Isn't it bad to exercise before bed?" It's not. A new report compiled the results of twenty-three studies and found that exercising 4 hours before bed actually helps you sleep, but they suggest avoiding vigorous exercise at least 1 hour before bedtime.[37]

This caution was suggested because of one study that examined the effects of running for 30 minutes at moderate or vigorous intensity 1 hour before bedtime.[38] They recruited active men who ran at both intensities on separate days. Matthew was one of them. The vigorous exercise elevated his heart rate **more than 25 beats per minute (bpm)** above baseline at bedtime, and it took him **14 minutes longer** than normal to fall asleep. In contrast, the moderate-intensity exercise did not elevate his heart rate at bedtime, and he fell asleep as fast as he normally did. Therefore, exercising before bedtime is not bad for sleep unless it is so intense that it elevates your heart rate more than 25 bpm above baseline.

How do you know if your heart rate is elevated? You can measure it yourself by placing the fingertips of your index and middle fingers on your wrist at the base of your thumb or on your neck just below your jawbone. Find your pulse. Now, count the number of beats for 1 minute. Count again and take the average. Note that your resting heart rate should be taken when seated after resting for about 20 minutes in a quiet, comfortable room that has minimal distraction.[39] At rest, the heart typically beats between 50 and 90 bpm, but that varies depending on your age, sex, and fitness level.[40]

Once you've established your resting heart rate, you can use that same method to check your heart rate at bedtime. If it's 25 bpm higher than at rest, it may take you longer to fall asleep.

Exercise for Insomnia and Anxiety

Exercise is not the only thing that can cause our heart to race before bed. Anxiety can elevate your heart rate to 138 bpm,[41] and people who have anxious thoughts just before bed take nearly **12 minutes longer** to fall asleep.[42] It can happen to anyone, even elite athletes, of whom over 60 percent admit to having difficulty falling asleep the night before a competition because they are preoccupied by their anxious thoughts about the big event.[43]

"This is something I struggle with on a nightly basis," Irene admits, and her insomnia symptoms are worse when she feels anxious. Can exercise help Irene? Yes! And because she struggles to fall asleep, exercising in the mornings or afternoons may work best for her brain time to "fall back" in line with real time.

Irene was willing to try but hadn't been exercising in years and wasn't sure how to start. After doing some research, we came up with a plan. We found several studies that demonstrated the benefits of exercise for insomnia across different protocols including yoga and tai chi,[44] but Irene liked the sound of this 6-week walking program with a gradual buildup.[45]

Irene's Exercise Program
Walk Outside Weekdays at 1 p.m.

Week 1	10 to 15 minutes	Easy pace
Week 2	15 to 20 minutes	A little faster
Week 3	20 to 25 minutes	A little faster still
Week 4	25 to 30 minutes	Brisk pace
Week 5	30 minutes	Brisk pace
Week 6	30 minutes	Brisk pace
...		

Irene showed the exercise plan to her doctor, who approved. Now, Irene was eager to get moving. After 11 years of chronic persistent insomnia, Irene was ready for a good night's sleep.

Just before setting out on her first walk, I told Irene about another study that used an exercise program like hers. The people tested had insomnia, and just 6 months of exercising reduced their insomnia symptoms. Irene wanted to be her own guinea pig to see if exercise would reduce her symptoms too. For the sake of time, I administered a modified version of the Insomnia Severity Index and asked her the following questions that she rated from zero (no, not applicable) to four (yes, very applicable):

1. Is it difficult for you to fall asleep?

2. Is it difficult for you to stay asleep?

3. Do you wake up too early?

4. How dissatisfied are you with your sleep?

5. Do your sleep problems interfere with your daily life?

6. Do other people notice your sleep problems?

7. How worried are you about your sleep problems?

Add the numbers from the answers to get your score. Higher scores indicate more severe insomnia. Based on the validated test,[46] a score of 15 or higher suggests clinical insomnia. Irene scored 16, indicating clinical insomnia of moderate severity. She confirmed that my quick assessment matched her doctor's prior diagnosis, and she was determined to see how low her symptoms would go with exercise.

After the initial 6 weeks, Irene continued walking for 6 months more.[47] Like clockwork, Irene was outside for her Wellness Walk at 1 p.m. sharp. We met up at the 6-month mark for her reassessment. Much to Irene's delight, her insomnia severity had dropped by *four* points and her insomnia symptoms were no longer clinical. "Incredible!" I exclaimed in amazement. But Irene wasn't surprised by the score. She had already noticed the change in her life. Since starting to exercise, she was falling asleep faster and sleeping more soundly, and all of this made her very happy.

Exercise and Sleeping More Soundly

Over those 6 months, Irene's fitness improved to the point that she was walking farther and faster than ever before. Although her consistency was helping her fall asleep faster, it was the intensity and duration of her walks that helped her sleep more soundly.[48] When it comes to deep sleep and exercise, more is better. And by more, I mean higher intensity and longer duration.

To understand why more exercise helps you sleep deeper, I need to introduce you to **adenosine** — nature's second sleeping aid.[49] Adenosine is a chemical found in all cells of the body, including the brain. It increases with every hour that you are active and awake and therefore provides a biological marker of how hard you have been working. The longer and harder you exercise, the more adenosine builds up during the day and the deeper you sleep at night.[50]

Your brain has a built-in sensor for detecting the rise of adenosine. When adenosine rises too high, the brain forces you to sleep.[51] Unlike melatonin, this sleeping aid works more like a battery than a clock, and **adenosine** levels indicate how much battery power your brain has used up. When your battery runs out of juice, you are forced to sleep no matter where you are or what time it is.

Dr. Aschoff's bunker experiment proved that people still sleep even when they are locked away in a dark cave with no sense of time.[52] Astronauts basically live in a bunker in the sky. During the Apollo 11 mission to the moon, there were times when the sun rose and set every 45 minutes and times when it didn't shine at all. Yet, according to the mission's record, Neil Armstrong still managed to sleep every night.[53] If you've ever worked a graveyard shift, you know this to be true. Your brain still sleeps every "night" even if it is most people's "day."[54] This is the power of adenosine. Dead battery trumps clock.

Like temperature, adenosine is under homeostatic control.[55] As adenosine nears dangerously high levels, the brain sends out a warning signal. "SOS! Time to sleep!" At that point, you may choose to ignore it. You may even try to suppress it.

"Another coffee?" asks the barista.

"Yes, please," you reply.

Until you've gone too far. Now, adenosine levels are too high. Your brain's SOS moves to its highest alert. "Enough is enough!" And suddenly, you're asleep . . . Seconds later, you wake up. The barista is staring at you, holding your coffee.

"What just happened?" you wonder. It turns out you were sleeping (err . . . *micro*sleeping). Hopefully, she didn't notice. She did. You probably shouldn't have stayed up all night finishing that project.

"I added an extra shot of espresso for you. It's on the house," she says and winks.

You blush. Too bad you're too tired to come up with anything clever to say. Doh!

HOW COFFEE KEEPS SLEEP AT BAY

You may cut back on sleep and think you can handle it with a little coffee. And there's no question that the barista is an absolute godsend after a poor night's sleep. But the coffee she serves only delays the inevitable. For adenosine to trigger an SOS, it must bind to its receptor, and caffeine blocks that receptor.[56] However, once the caffeine wears off and the receptor is freed up, adenosine levels may already be too high and, without warning, you're asleep.

Exercise Promotes Deeper Sleep

Here's the bottom line: Exercise helps drain the brain's battery during the day for a deeper sleep at night.

Deep sleep is exactly what you need to pay off your so-called **sleep debt**, which refers to the accumulated sleep that you've missed.[57] Chronically undersleeping causes you to accumulate sleep debt, making you feel sleepy when you should be awake. And be warned, a small sleep debt can accumulate into a larger sleep debt very quickly. Remember Randy Gardner, the teen who stayed awake for 11 days? By the end of the experiment, he had accumulated a sleep debt of 88 hours. Although you and I may never stay awake for that long, we can accumulate a similar sleep debt by restricting our sleep for just 2 hours a night over 44 nights, and that is not good for our health.[58]

Consider the case of **fatal familial insomnia (FFI)**, a rare but deadly sleep disorder that prevents people from sleeping deeply.[59] It's like insomnia on steroids! At best, the brain sneaks in a little shut-eye but nothing deep. In fact, once FFI strikes, which is typically after the age of 40, the individual will **never sleep deeply again**. Fortunately, FFI is rare, but it does run in families. Francesco's family calls it the family curse. Now that Francesco is 40, he prays that he won't get the curse. Otherwise, he'll be dead before his 42nd birthday. Dead! That's how vital deep sleep is.

Through the night, our sleep depth varies depending on the speed and synchrony of the brain's activity. When we are active and awake, the brain works lightning fast.[60] Its rhythms desynchronize to move the body and focus the mind. At this rate, the brain's battery drains quickly. After about 16 hours, its charge is low and it's time for bed.

STAGE 1: LIGHT SLEEP
A drowsy state that lasts only a few minutes. The brain slows down from the busy day, and its rhythms start to synchronize.

STAGE 2: DEEPER SLEEP
Your consciousness fades as the brain slows and synchronizes even more, except for the occasional bursts of brain activity known as **spindles** that interrupt the brain's regular rhythm but not your sleep. In fact, you need spindles to go deeper. Most people stay at this stage for 10 to 25 minutes before going deeper. People with FFI lack spindles, so this is as deep as

they go.[61] Unfortunately, this means that their brain only recharges a little but not a lot.

STAGE 3: SLOW WAVE SLEEP (SWS)

Completely unconscious and oblivious to the world around you. Your brain slows down to a near halt, dominated by delta waves. These big slow delta waves are fully synchronized, like big surf waves that virtually wash your brain clean.[62] They are what make sleep so refreshing! Deep sleep is also a perfect time to recharge, and the more time we spend in this stage, the faster we pay back our sleep debt. The first cycle of SWS usually lasts 20 to 40 minutes, though SWS lasts longer after a day of exercise.[63] More exercise equals more SWS.[64]

REM SLEEP

After SWS, the brain transitions into a paradoxical stage of sleep called **rapid eye movement (REM) sleep**. The sleeping brain's rhythms become lightning fast and desynchronize as if it were awake. The body is paralyzed, except for the eyes, which move rapidly (hence the name). This is when we **dream** our most vivid, complex, and emotional dreams.[65] Though your first episode of REM lasts mere minutes before heading back into SWS, the brain continues to cycle between SWS and REM. It completes four to six cycles a night. Each cycle lasts about 90 minutes and contains less SWS and more REM as the night progresses. As we pay back our sleep debt and recharge the brain's battery, adenosine levels return to baseline and our need for deep sleep decreases. **Exercising more during the day helps us pay back our sleep debt faster so that we wake up feeling more refreshed and recharged.**

Moving more to sleep better is especially important as we get older, because SWS declines with **age**. Some older adults only spend 5 percent of their total sleep time in SWS and never feel well rested.[66] With less big delta surf to wash their brains clean, toxic residues build up to form brain plaques.[67] This may be why poor sleep increases the risk of Alzheimer's disease.[68] Fortunately, aerobic and resistance exercise can improve sleep quality in middle-aged and older adults with sleep problems to remedy this.[69]

But as modern-day life continues to chip away at our precious bedtime, everyone could stand to bank a few extra hours of sleep for those days when you just can't get enough. The first study to test whether we could **bank sleep** recruited twenty-four young adults, including Ella and Haley.[70] Prior to a week of restricted sleep for 3 hours a night, the women were assigned to two different sleep conditions:

1. Ella was in the **extended sleep** group and slept for 10 hours a night the week before the week of restricted sleep.

2. Haley was in the **habitual sleep** group and slept for 7 hours a night the week before the week of restricted sleep.

Banking those extra 21 hours of sleep saved Ella big time! During the week of restricted sleep, both women performed poorly on a vigilance test, but Haley performed worse. Also, it took Haley a lot longer to recover. Even after 5 full nights of sleep, Haley was still not performing her best, whereas Ella had bounced back quickly. She was almost back to being her best self after just 1 night of good sleep.

Because exercise naturally extends and deepens sleep, you can use exercise to aid in building your **sleep savings account** to help you bank sleep for when you need it the most.

A Caution on Using Alcohol to Alleviate Insomnia

Some people self-medicate with alcohol. Although alcohol is a sedative that slows down the brain, does a nightcap actually help you sleep? The truth is, having a drink before bed can help you fall asleep faster and sleep more soundly — but you pay for it later.[71] Alcohol disrupts the second half of your sleep, making you REM deficient.

"What's the big deal about missing a few dreams?" you wonder.

Well, it turns out that REM's dreams are not merely for our sleeping brain's entertainment. REM helps us contextualize emotional memories so they are less emotionally distressing.[72] This may be why my mom always says, "Go to bed; you'll feel better in the morning." And she's right, I do, unless I've been drinking. Then I feel worse. When REM sleep is disrupted, we are more likely to be haunted by our emotional memories that seem disproportionally scary. It happens in insomnia[73] and PTSD[74] and could contribute to an alcoholic's anxiety.[75]

How much alcohol is too much? Although there is no formal guideline, light consumption of one to two standard drinks appears to be less harmful than heavy consumption of more than four standard drinks.[76]

Can exercise help? Although exercise can help addicts ease their anxiety during recovery (see Chapter 4), it does not seem to protect us against the negative effects of alcohol on sleep.[77] So, skip the drink and go for a workout. It will help you fall asleep faster and sleep more deeply throughout the entire night.

And on that note, it really is quite late. Time for me to get some shut-eye. What's on my to-do list for tomorrow? Definitely exercise. Right at the top. My sleep has been especially deep lately, as I begin the final stretch of my full Ironman training. The good news is you don't have to train that intensely to sleep well. The Good Night's Sleep Workout on page 136 will help you add a little more intensity and duration to your exercise program — the boost you need for a better sleep. Sleep well, sweet dreams.

The Good Night's Sleep Workout

REFERENCE: Chapter 6   **NEURO FIX:** Reset the brain's clock
MINDSET: Consistent effort   **LEVEL:** Advanced

MON	TUES	WED	THURS	FRI	SAT	SUN
Wellness Run	Rise and Shine	Wellness Run	Sprints for Shut-Eye	Wellness Run	Sound Sleeper	

WELLNESS WALK-TO-RUN

Warm up with a 5-minute Wellness Walk. Walk or run for 30 minutes at a comfortably challenging pace at the same time every day. Morning is best if you're struggling to fall asleep at night.

Ready to take the next step? Run 5 minutes longer every week.

RISE AND SHINE

Warm up with a 5-minute Wellness Walk, then complete exercises 1 to 8 for the prescribed repetitions. Take a 30-second mindful break. Focus on your breathing. Repeat.

ORDER	EXERCISE	REPETITIONS	PICTURED
1	Front Plank	30 seconds	Page 175
2	Supine Hip Lifts (single leg)	10 reps per side	Page 198
3	Split Squats	10 reps per side	Page 194
4	Pushups	10 reps	Page 185
5	Bicycles	10 reps per side	Page 169
6	Kneeling Donkey Kicks	10 reps per side	Page 180
7	Lateral Raises	10 reps	Page 182
8	Jumping Jacks	30 seconds	Page 178
	Mindful Break	30 seconds	

Ready to take the next step? Increase your repetitions to 15 reps and 40 seconds. Repeat the exercises a third time.

SPRINTS FOR SHUT-EYE

Warm up with a 10-minute Soothing Cycle (page 66), then go as fast as you can go for as long as you can. Try for 20 seconds. Take a 2-minute Soothing Cycle break, then repeat six times. Cool down with a 10-minute Wellness Walk. Complete at least 1 hour before bed so that your heart rate has time to recover.

Ready to take the next step? Add another repeat each week.

THE SOUND SLEEPER

Warm up with a 5-minute Wellness Walk, then complete exercises 1 to 8 for the prescribed repetitions. Take a 30-second mindful break. Focus on your breathing. Repeat.

ORDER	EXERCISE	REPETITIONS	PICTURED
1	Side Plank	30 seconds	Page 190
2	Superman (alternating)	10 reps per side	Page 197
3	Squats	10 reps per side	Page 195
4	Pushups	10 reps	Page 185
5	Row (single arm)	10 reps per side	Page 187
6	Hip Openers	10 reps per side	Page 177
7	Dead Bugs	10 reps per side	Page 173
8	Skaters	30 seconds	Page 193
	Mindful Break	30 seconds	

Ready to take the next step? Increase your repetitions to 15 reps and 40 seconds. Repeat the exercises a third time.

7

STAYING FOCUSED, BEING CREATIVE, AND STICKING TO IT

Not all marathons are won at the finish line.

— THE TERRY FOX FOUNDATION

H OORAY! YOU'RE WELL on your way.
Fitness goal in check.
Life goals. Check. Check.
The journey has not always been easy.
At times, it's been hard to stay focused, but you've endured.
How? Because you're stronger now, and it's no secret why.
Exercise is your medicine. A remedy that has healed you in so many ways.
You're smiling more.
Craving less.
Remembering lots.
Sleeping well.
And now that you're really moving, it's easier for you to stay focused.
You get things done faster.

Creative solutions come to you effortlessly.

Exercise has unlocked your brain's greatest potential. Enjoy those moments of genius. You've earned them!

So, let's celebrate! After all, it's taken us years to get here.

Sure, we started out with a goal in mind and set our eyes on that prize.

But this is a lifelong journey. Pace yourself. Enjoy the experience. Make each moment count. This is what it takes to persevere all the way to the end.

In this final chapter, you will learn how to optimize exercise to stay focused and be creative. Then I will touch on getting into flow, understanding the value of grit, appreciating the exercise experience, and continuing even when the going gets tough.

STAYING FOCUSED WHEN IT MATTERS MOST

It was a new year, a new decade, and I had set my New Year's resolution on completing a full Ironman. This would mark the end of my 3-year journey from frailty to fitness that strengthened my body and mind. I was almost there. The race was set for August 23, 2020. My coach had created a great plan to get me ready. All I had to do was execute it. Fortunately, all my training had helped to keep me focused. In fact, this is one of the most desirable benefits that exercise bestows on the brain.

Great Minds

The brain is most revered for its incredible ability to think and create. These skills are governed by its most evolved region, the prefrontal cortex.[1] Our expansive prefrontal cortex is what separates us from all other animals. It's why we don't just react to the world; we interact with it. It allows us to reflect on what we've learned from the past, imagine what it could be like in the future, and set plans in motion to make our thoughts a reality. Just look at all the incredible things that we have accomplished.

But we don't always think great, do we? Sometimes we see things as possibilities. Other times we see those same things as roadblocks. In Chapter 6, we learned how sleeplessness makes it harder for us to think clearly. But the truth is that all ailments discussed in this book impact our ability to think great. People with **anxiety** and **depression** have diffi-culty concentrating — so much so that it's actually part of the diagnosis.[2] **Addiction** disrupts the brain's ability to regulate emotions and impulses, and this makes it harder for us to make good decisions.[3] **Older adults** struggle to ignore distractions and organize their thoughts, which can be very confusing.[4] To compensate for our lack of focus, we may narrow our minds in the hopes that it will help, but it only makes it more difficult for us to understand another's point of view. As we struggle to analyze the situation, develop an effective plan, and communicate that plan to others, it becomes more challenging for us to lead.

Part of the problem is we've put all our eggs in one basket. *Cogito, ergo sum.* I think, therefore I am. Some people love this quote, but I absolutely hate it. I blame René Descartes, the quote maker, and his theory of mind-body dualism for creating the predicament we're in. "Mind versus body!" he declared. And it's no secret who we've sided with. Just look at how much time we've taken away from the body and given to the mind. "With good intention, mind you," reminds the mind. "After all, mental pursuits are important for productivity." Yes, but spending all that time in one's head is actually counterproductive.

Descartes was wrong! The mind and body are not separate but *depen-dent* on each other. We need to move to think great. That's the bottom line.

Here's the scenario: You're in the middle of a meeting. There's a dead-line at work, and you're leading the project. Today's briefing will help you get that project done. Your boss is telling you exactly what the client wants. "It's important that you include these things in the final project," she emphasizes. You nod. But wait . . . did you actually hear what she said? You didn't. Oh, no! "Um, do you mind repeating that last bit?" you ask. She's annoyed but repeats it anyway. It's very important that you get this.

"Hmm . . . what should we have for lunch?" asks your mind mindlessly.

"How can you be daydreaming at a time like this!" you scold as your boss continues and you realize you've missed it again. Doh! Hopefully, someone else on your team was in the right mind to hear it.

What happened to you in that meeting? It's called **mind wandering**,[5] and it's the exact opposite mindset that you needed to be in to focus on what your boss was saying. You see, the brain is made up of a collection of networks, or different brain regions, that work together. Mind wandering is governed by the default mode network; this is **vacation mode**. "Sounds great; I could use a vacation," you admit. But the reality is that your brain spends a lot of time on vacation, using your imagination to travel back and forth in time. Where to? It doesn't really matter. What matters is that you're *waaay* off task. The most obvious off-taskers are talking, texting, doodling, and fidgeting. The least obvious off-taskers are stealthily still; they are not talking, texting, doodling, or fidgeting, but they are not listening either. When it comes to focused thinking, all off-taskers suffer equally. Get back to work!

Work mode is governed by a different brain network, called the executive control network. As you can imagine, work mode requires more effort than vacation mode, and when the brain gets tired, it automatically switches over to vacation mode.[6]

To think great, we rely on the coordinated efforts of three executive functions:[7]

1. **Working memory:** Working memory displays all the thoughts you have in mind and lets you manipulate them. Its space is limited, akin to a 7-inch screen, which means that its contents are constantly changing. To open a new "file," it must close another. Some files are saved (remembered), but others are not (forgotten). Both work mode and vacation mode use working memory to present their ideas.

2. **Inhibitory control:** Work mode can't have any distractions, so it suppresses vacation mode to keep you *focused*. This is the function of inhibitory control and the main reason work mode is so exhausting.

3. **Mental flexibility:** This is important for combining ideas from work and play for *creative thinking*. Switching between work mode and play mode is controlled by a third brain network called the **salience network**, which works like a remote control to change the channel.

Some people have a larger working memory, more inhibitory control, and greater mental flexibility than others; this makes it easier for them to think, work, and manage their daily lives.[8] Exercise enhances executive functions,[9] which means **you can train for a sharper brain!**

Boost Your Brain Power with Exercise

A short movement break is all it takes to refuel your brain so you can get back to work.

After exercising, your brain is as sharp as it can possibly be. Bathed in blood sugar and oxygen, your prefrontal cortex performs its suite of executive functions with absolute precision. This creates a window of opportunity to fine-tune your thinking.

A little goes a long way! My lab has shown that short **5-minute exercise breaks** are better than no breaks or sedentary breaks when it comes to staying on task.[10] We used high-intensity calisthenics like the Neuro Fix on page 162, but light or moderate movements would work well too because within the first 15 minutes of exercise, light, moderate, and hard intensities all yield the same boost in oxygenated blood flow to the prefrontal cortex, though more oxygenated blood rushes in the longer and more vigorously you exercise.[11]

For a light exercise break, try the Opener on page 18.

For a moderate exercise break, try the Uplifter on page 65.

For a vigorous exercise break, try the Neuro Fix on page 162.

"Can I do that in a meeting?" you wonder.

Hmm . . . probably not. You could stand up and move to the back of the room. A little goes a long way. But it's probably best to prepare ahead of time. Incorporate exercise as part of your meeting prep. The boost you get from exercising can keep you focused for up to 2 hours afterward.[12]

Academic Performance and Exercise for Children

When a teacher, Ms. Evelyn Baker, read about our research, she wondered whether exercise breaks would help her fourth grade class stay focused; they had been very disruptive lately. Ms. Baker tested it. In between lessons, she led her class in a 5-minute movement break including high knees, sit stands, and jumping jacks. She was so pleased with the results that she started incorporating movement into her lessons too.[13] She calls them **energizers**: where the kids act like lions when learning about lions or jump out the solution to a math problem, $1 + 1 = 2$ jumping jacks. She couldn't believe the difference in her students. The exercise breaks made them less disruptive, less distracted, and better learners. The other teachers started to notice and wanted in on her secret. Ms. Baker gladly shared, and soon the whole school was moving more.

Then, worries started to circulate. Some parents wondered whether the school was spending enough time on the academic content. One mother was outright against it. "I don't want my child to fall behind academically!" She was the president of the PTA and promptly called a meeting. They invited me to speak.

"It's quality over quantity," I explained. "Research shows that students in active classrooms learn just as much as students in inactive classrooms but in less time, and active classrooms result in more durable learning. You may even see a better grade on your child's report card."

"And the students love it!" added Ms. Baker.

"And so do the teachers!" added another teacher, while all the teachers nodded vigorously in agreement.

I encouraged the parents to try it out for themselves: "Take a 5-minute exercise break at least once throughout your workday, and see if you notice a difference in how you think and feel."

A week went by, and I got a call from the PTA president. Much to her amazement, the exercise breaks worked! At work, between meetings, she snuck in a few flights of stairs, and the movement made her feel calmer and more focused. Most importantly, she was able to get all her work done in less time. She called to tell me that she's 100 percent on board! She was so on board that she wondered whether in-class activity was enough: "Should my child be doing more activity after school? Will it have the same benefit?"

I tell her, "Yes! Children who are more physically active are more focused during class and perform better academically."[14]

"Is more always better?" she asked. "How little time can we devote to this? Busy parents need to know."

The Right Dose of Extracurricular Exercise for Children

The World Health Organization recommends that children and youth accumulate at least 60 minutes of moderate to vigorous physical activity every day.[15] It does a body good! But what about the brain?

My lab answered this question in a recent study, and it turns out the brain gets away with much less.[16] We asked a diverse group of 31,000 students in elementary and high school two questions. The first asked about their physical activity level: "Over the past 7 days, on how many days did you engage in physical activity for at least 60 minutes that increased your heart rate and made you out of breath?" The second question asked about their academic achievement: "Based on your report card, how are you doing in the following subjects: language (reading, writing, oral communication), mathematics, and overall?"

Busy parents will be happy to hear that there is a **minimum dose** of physical activity needed for academic achievement, but it differs depending on the child's age.

For elementary students:

- One to two days were better than no days.
- More days were better.
- Seven days were best.

For high school students:

- Three to four days were the minimum.
- There was no additional benefit of adding more days.

In that same study, we also discovered *how* physical activity improved academic achievement. Students who were more physically active achieved better academically because they were less inattentive and hyperactive in class. Not a big shocker, but it hints at the real reason physical activity works to improve academic performance — because it enhances executive functions.

For children struggling with attention deficit hyperactivity disorder (ADHD), physical activity helps alleviate their cognitive, behavioral, and physical symptoms.[17] Abby's son Aiden has ADHD, and his daily dose of physical activity is a must. In elementary school, Aiden had physical education every day, and she noticed the benefits right away: "His ability to focus drastically improved. His brain was so much sharper. It was almost like the activity got rid of his restlessness." But when Aiden transitioned into high school, he lost his daily dose of exercise and his restlessness returned. Abby started getting notes from Aiden's teachers about his disruptive behavior. That's when she made the connection: His brain needed exercise to think. She encouraged Aiden to work out with her every morning before school, and once they started, the notes stopped. Children and adults with ADHD have difficulty focusing because their prefrontal cortex lacks the vital nutrients it needs. It's deficient in blood flow and dopamine.[18] Exercise has the potential to correct this deficit by altering the same neural systems as Ritalin and Adderall but without the unwanted side effects.[19]

Although Ms. Baker was an early adopter of active classrooms, more teachers are recognizing the benefits of movement for learning. Based on the latest research, every school should have pedal desks, a stationary bike, or at least an open space at the back of the class where students can move. One study found that about 20 minutes of moderate-intensity aerobic exercise was enough to boost executive functions for at least 1 hour afterward.[20] What's more, the boost in executive functions from exercise is seen for all children, not just the ones with ADHD.[21]

Exercise and Enhanced Focus

Come to think of it, we could all benefit from a little more movement throughout the day. That's because exercise benefits executive functions across the lifespan.[22] Of all the executive functions that benefit from exercise, researchers have focused on inhibitory control,[23] which seems to benefit the most,[24] though I suspect this is an artifact of the simplified exercises we do in the lab.

Here's my confession: Exercising in my lab is not fun. Don't expect to walk into a high-end health club. There's no sauna. No towel service. Sometimes, we don't even give you the choice of equipment. We simply put you on the treadmill (err . . . dread-mill) and ask you to exercise alone in a quiet, temperature-controlled room while staring at a blank wall. Try doing that for 30 minutes! You'll likely spend the entire time trying to *stop* yourself from thinking about how boring the workout is. "How many more minutes do I have left?" you ask. "Are you sure it's only been five?" It's not just a physical workout, it's a mental workout too.

When you exercise this way, you're essentially doing two things at once: You're exercising your body and you're exercising your mind, or more specifically, your inhibitory control. If you're lucky enough to be selected for one of our training programs, you'll train that way three

times a week for 6 months. When it's all said and done, you will be physically fitter and mentally stronger too. Think of all the hours you've just
spent suppressing boredom. Now, you're an inhibiting machine.

Impulses? No problem.

Temptations? Bring them on!

Distractions? Irrelevant.

That may sound great, but there is a problem. Unfortunately, you've
flexed only one of your executive functions. Everything was so focused
and regulated that you didn't use your mental flexibility at all. This
can be especially frustrating for children with autism like Asher, who
needs help with mental flexibility rather than focus.[25] My lab and others have found that Asher's executive functions improve more with circuit training than treadmill training.[26] Table tennis[27] and basketball[28]
work well too. Critically, all of these activities provide the opportunity
for the brain to flex its mental flexibility, which we all need to enhance
our creativity.

EXERCISING FOR CREATIVITY

Being a great thinker is not just about being focused. It's about being
creative too. When we think creatively, we think outside of the box and
use our imagination to create novel and appropriate ideas. Guess which
brain network is best at this? That's right, it's time for a vacation!

Most of my creative victories are celebrated *privately*. A scheduling
problem at home ingeniously fixed. "Mom for the win!" I cheer and give
myself a subtle yet affirmative nod to the mirror.

Other creative victories are celebrated *publicly*. A brilliantly executed
play made by a world-class athlete. "Bravo!" we all cheer. Public creative
victories are much more glamorous and spectacular than private ones,
and perhaps not surprisingly, the majority of research on exercise and
creativity has focused on sport. Therefore, this section will be the "sports
section" of my book. For all of you nonathletes out there (my former self
included), keep an open mind, because all of these results can be applied
to enhance your life both on and off the field. And make no mistake,
the brain uses the same networks to come up with a creative solution
whether that win is private or public.

One of my favorite athletes of all time is Wayne Gretzky, one of the greatest hockey players to ever play the game. But he almost didn't make the cut. Why? Back then, the players were big, and the game was aggressive. It was not suitable for a small player like Gretzky. So, he created an entirely new way of playing the game — inside the rules but outside the box. His play was creative and unpredictable. It was about skill rather than aggressiveness. And he won games, lots of them, earning nearly 1,000 more points than any other hockey player to ever play the game. It was Gretzky's creative thinking that made him great. And it's your creative thinking that makes you great too.

How creative are you? One way to measure your creativity is by using the Alternative Uses Test, which assesses your ability to think *divergently*. Your task? Set a timer for 3 minutes, and list as many unique uses for a *paper clip* that you can think of. Ready, set, go! . . . And done!

Now, count the number of unique responses you generated. One study found that the average number of unique responses generated was ten, but people's responses ranged from one to twenty-six.[29] More unique responses equals more creativity.

Who are the most creative people among us? Artists and scientists[30] and . . . athletes. Yes, athletes, but it depends on the sport. One study examined the creativity of 208 world-class athletes from a wide range of sports including artistic, combat, invasion, net, and racing.[31] Their creativity was assessed using a divergent thinking task, similar to the test above, and their creativity was measured in three ways:

1. Creative fluency, the *total* number of ideas generated.

2. Originality, the number of *unique* ideas generated.

3. Flexibility, the number of ideas related to *different categories*.

The most skilled athletes had the greatest creative fluency, originality, and flexibility, demonstrating a direct connection between sport performance and creativity.

Which sports produced the most creative athletes? It may surprise you. It wasn't artistic sports but net and combat sports. Why? Because cultivating a creative mind depends on *how* we train.

In **artistic** sports (figure skating, gymnastics, synchronized swimming), the athlete memorizes a series of predefined steps. Although coming up with these steps may be creative, the training itself is prescribed, predictable, and planned. As the athlete physically trains, her brain trains too. But with these sports, her brain is flexing its inhibitory control the most. And because of this, she ends up becoming less mentally flexible.

Contrast this with **net and combat sports** (badminton, racquetball, volleyball, fencing): The athlete learns to instinctively react to the ever-changing actions of their opponent. Training is more impulsive, unpredictable, and improvised. As the athlete physically trains, his brain trains too. But with these sports, his brain is flexing its cognitive flexibility the most. And because of this, he ends up becoming more creative. **Therefore, by training your body to move more creatively, you train your mind to think more creatively.**

"Umm, what about us nonathletic folk?" my friend Kathleen wonders.

"Fortunately, you don't have to train like an Olympian to get your creative juices flowing." Here are some less intensive alternatives:

- Walking for about 10 minutes at a self-selected pace.[32]
- Performing hatha yoga for 20 minutes.[33]
- Jogging, swimming, biking, or stair climbing for 30 minutes.[34]

To Maximize Your Creative Thinking, You Need to Cross-Train!

No matter the exercise options you gravitate toward, be careful not to spend too much time on one activity, or you may inadvertently train yourself into a funk. Of course, mastery of any subject matter requires focused practice, but to a point. Beyond that point, you get less bang for your *training* buck. You also risk getting stuck in a conventional rut — the dreaded state of **functionally fixedness**. It can happen to the best of us, even world-class athletes. For example, athletes who train exclusively in one sport are *less creative* than those who train in more than one sport, even if they play the other sport for fun.[35]

Worst of all, being too focused causes you to miss other things, sometimes important things that may be right in front of your eyes. Psychologists call it **inattentional blindness**, and the cheekiest demonstration of it involves a basketball game and a dancing gorilla.[36] Let's cast you as the participant. You're instructed to watch a video of six basketball players. There are two teams with three players each. Both teams have a basketball and are passing it to the players on their team. Your job? Count the number of passes made by one team while ignoring the passes made by the other team. It's harder than it sounds because the six players are haphazardly positioned around a small circle and the balls cross paths.

The researcher presses "Play" to start the video. You flex your strong inhibitory control and start to count. At the end of the video, you provide your count. Seventeen?

Correct! But did you see the gorilla? He must be kidding. He's not. Confused, you play the video again and there's the gorilla, smack dab in the middle of the game, and he's doing a little dance. A dance! You are shocked to have missed such a spectacle. But don't worry, you're not alone. Half the people who watched the video failed to see it too. It's a good thing you were in an experiment and not in real life. How bad would it be to miss something so blatant?

Although the brain can process many things at once, the mind cannot. It has one track. Your working memory limits the contents of your mind to its itty-bitty 7-inch screen. When two things are competing for your attention at once, you have to choose. You can only focus on one thing at a time. Here's the play: The researcher-turned-coach instructs you, "If the player defending comes at you, then deceive him with a feint. Otherwise, take the shot." The game unfolds, and you end up taking a shot, just as the coach instructed, but you miss and it costs your team the game.

Your teammates are mad and question your play. "Why didn't you pass the ball to Evans?" It turns out, Evans was wide open and in much better scoring position than you. You didn't pass it to Evans because you didn't see him. You didn't see Evans because you were so focused on the coach's instructions. But you are not alone. When overtly coached, the vast majority of players don't see the unmarked man.[37] When not overtly coached, the vast majority of players see the unmarked man, and instead of taking the shot, they get the ball to Evans and win the game. **When our mind is not full of instructions, it has room to play with new ideas that can lead to great discoveries.**

Can you imagine how this would play out at work or home? Someone instructs you to do a task in a very specific way and then watches closely to make sure you execute every step perfectly. I guarantee you'll make a mistake. Why? Because it's hard to think great when your mind is full of instructions and anxiety. We need to give each other the opportunity to play creatively with new ideas, regardless of the outcome. Only then can we be truly innovative.

A Case for Letting Kids Play

Gretzky believes overcoaching is hockey's problem. Scoring has been at an all-time low. Is the game broken? No, but according to Gretzky, the coaching is. Gretzky remembers the good old days, when he and his friends would go down to the frozen pond, divide into teams, throw the puck down, and play. Could today's youth do that? Gretzky is doubtful. He thinks they wouldn't know what to do because everything has to be lined up for them. Everything has to be regimented. And we've got to get away from that.

Here's a case in Gretzky's point. Road hockey is a Canadian tradition. No coaches. No parents. Just kids with sticks, a net, and a puck. The city of Toronto, Canada's largest, tried to ban road hockey. They even threatened to fine kids if caught playing in the streets. Fortunately for the sake of Canada's future innovation, this ruling was overturned. In fact, there is a direct link between the amount of free play a child does between the ages of 5 and 14 years old and their creative potential as adults. Not just in hockey but in life. A study measured the creativity of nearly 100 adults, then asked them about the type and amount of physical activity they did as children. The activities included structured sport and unstructured free play.[38]

It turns out that the ratio of **structured to unstructured activities** a child does predicts their creative potential in adulthood.

- **70:30** was the ratio of the **least creative** adults, who spent the majority of their childhood in organized sports.
- **50:50** was the ratio of the **most creative** adults, who split their time during childhood evenly between organized sports and free play.

The optimal weekly dose of free play for creativity is **2 or more hours a week**. Free time to play gives kids the opportunity to try out new ways of doing things that may or may not work—but that's irrelevant. And more to the point, isn't it always the most epic fails that make for the greatest stories? That's how kids learn. That's how we all learn.

CAN EXERCISE ENHANCE BOTH
FOCUS AND CREATIVITY AT THE SAME TIME?

Yes, you can train to enhance both focus *and* creativity, but your training program must include **unpredictability**, **cross-training**, and **play**. For those of you who are just starting out, the mere act of exercising offers everything that you need. For those of you who are already active, you will need to change things up. Try out a new workout (might I suggest the Achiever on page 161). If you're already doing cardio, add strength exercises. If you are already doing strength exercises, add cardio. Infuse novelty into your current plan by including elements of surprise. Try exercising outdoors or take an unfamiliar route. Pick up a new sport or activity and play it with friends just for fun. Most importantly, find the mode of exercising that feels most like play to you. The payoff will be great!

How great? Ever heard of flow?

ALL ABOUT FLOW, GRIT, AND
FOCUSING ON THE EXPERIENCE

Getting to Flow

Flow is an effortless state of seemingly superhuman ability where you are fully immersed in the task, captivated by the moment, pushed to the absolute limits of body or mind in pursuit of a worthwhile goal.[39] These are your moments of pure genius!

Flow happens when the brain has what it needs to be both focused (work mode) and creative (vacation mode) *at the same time*. Creatively[40] cross-training with exercise can help make this happen! The brain power you typically need to switch between work mode and vacation mode is freed up, and you save in three ways:

1. Pushed outside of your comfort zone, the task is challenging but doable. Noradrenaline infuses your prefrontal cortex, intensifying your focus.[41] Work mode engages *effortlessly,* and you save brain power.

2. It feels incredible to perform so well. Dopamine activates your default mode network, but it's not pulling you away from the task at hand because nothing is more interesting than this (not even a vacation).[42] Work mode spends less energy inhibiting vacation mode, and you save more brain power.

3. You can't believe how well you're performing. Work mode and vacation mode are not competing, they're collaborating.[43] This gives your working memory full access to your entire repertoire of knowledge, skill set, and experience. No need to switch back and forth, and you save even more brain power.

What do you do with all that extra brain power? You do extraordinary things both on and off the field.

How to Exercise for Unstoppable Perseverance

Flow is the ultimate experience, but it requires a lot of hard work to get there, and the journey will not always be easy. The best of the best knows what it takes to make it all the way to the end. Now, I know what you're thinking: "Aren't the best of the best just innately endowed?" Sure, many world-class athletes are gifted with special physical traits, but it takes much more than those traits to be great. Consider Michael Phelps, for example, whose size-14 feet are affixed with double-jointed ankles; they are more like flippers than feet. But take away Phelps's grit, and he's just a regular guy with unusually large and flexible feet rather than the most decorated Olympian of all time.

What's **grit**? It is a term reserved for the most dedicated among us.[44] The people who have the courage to follow their convictions. The conscientiousness to make sure the job is done right. The perseverance needed to pursue a goal in spite of any difficulties. The resiliency to rebound quickly thereafter. Confidence, passion, and purpose. People with grit are simply the best!

How to Become Your Grittiest Self

You've probably heard of the **10,000-hour rule**, popularized by Malcolm Gladwell. According to that rule, it takes 10,000 hours of practice to master any complex task. I did the math: 10,000 hours works out to about 20 hours a week for *10 years!* Fortunately, the 10,000-hour rule is not true. The truth is you may need *less* time. You may need *more* time. It all depends on *how* you train.

Tim Ferriss, the author of *The 4-Hour Workweek* and an efficiency guru, thinks he could master just about anything in a year or less, and he's probably right. I'm guessing he already knows how to leverage his brain's maximum learning capacity. The problem with the 10,000-hour rule is that it doesn't specify *how* to train, and this is key. Take middle-distance runners, for example. Their races range from 800 to 3,000 meters. These distances are extremely difficult to train for. They're longer than a sprint but shorter than a marathon. The best of the best must have great endurance and great speed. Specialized training is required. It's less about quantity and more about quality. In fact, elite middle-distance runners train just as much as their nonelite counterparts but devote more time to strength exercises and technical drills.[45] They're not training longer, just smarter.

Maybe you don't want to be the best of the best. (*Gasp!* Just kidding, it's okay.) Maybe you just want to be you — only healthier. That's definitely a goal worth striving for. Fortunately, the 10,000-hour rule doesn't apply here either. In fact, it doesn't apply to any goal. **Deliberate practice** can help you reach any goal faster.[46] How? By identifying something specific that you want to improve and then tailoring your training to improve that particular skill until it seamlessly integrates into your performance. Use deliberate practice to enhance your performance in sports and life.

The only downside is that deliberate practice is more intense than regular practice and requires much more brain power. Good thing you've got all that extra brain power built up from cross-training. You're going to need it! Be prepared to have your working memory, inhibitory control, and cognitive flexibility taxed to the max. All of your executive functions are needed to lay the foundation for your **stick-to-itiveness** — the dogged determination you'll need to stay steadfastly focused on your goal in spite of the endless distractions and temptations you'll face over the next months, even years. That's a long time to maintain such a high level of focus.

Fortunately, sticking to your fitness goal will get easier the longer you persevere. Why? Remember, exercise strengthens your executive functions, which, in turn, will make it easier for you to plan your workouts, creatively fit them into your busy schedule, and convince your lazy brain to get up off the couch and go to the gym. It's a virtuous cycle!

Here's where your strong inhibitory control pays off the most. It gifts you with incredible self-control that increases the likelihood that you'll make it past the first few months of any new fitness program. This was demonstrated by a recent study that examined the importance of self-control in achieving a health goal. They tracked a group of eighty-six people at the start of a new weight loss program.[47] The group was mostly women, 18 to 60 years old and keenly intent on losing weight, who had enrolled in a 12-week intervention to eat healthy and exercise. The participants met as a group once per week to discuss strategies, but otherwise they were on their own.

Some of the participants were more successful than others. Those who lost the most weight had the **highest self-control**. They also attended more meetings, consumed fewer calories, and exercised more. Their stronger self-control endowed them with the brain power they needed to make the necessary (yet difficult) changes to their diet and exercise. That said, this intervention was only 12 weeks, and the people with higher self-control came into the study that way, so they had a head start.

Can You Train for a More Health-Conscious Brain?

Yes! This was demonstrated by a recent study that recruited older women, 65 to 75 years old, whose executive functions were low to begin with because of their age.[48] The intervention had two parts: Part 1 involved 12 months of supervised exercise. Participants met once or twice per week at the gym with a fitness instructor who led them through a 60-minute workout. The workouts varied depending on their group.

- **The strength-training group** engaged in challenging resistance exercises that got more difficult as the months progressed. Over the 12 months, this group got physically and mentally stronger.
- **The control group** engaged in stretching and toning exercises that did not get more difficult as the months progressed. As expected, over the 12 months, this group did not get physically or mentally stronger.

⇨ Why have a control group like this? To isolate the true benefit of the strength-training exercises while controlling the
participants' dedication and socialization.

Part 2 consisted of 12 months of unsupervised exercise;[49] the participants were encouraged to continue exercising on their own. Unfortunately, most participants stopped exercising soon after the study was
over. This is typical and underscores how difficult it can be to exercise
on your own.

But Sonya was different. She was a participant in the strength-training
group. By the end of Part 1, her executive functions had substantially
improved, and this helped her stay physically active long after the supervised part of the study was over. In fact, Sonya was still exercising more
than a year later.

How Can We Get More People Past That 1-Year Mark?

It's a lifelong process. Of course, no one starts an exercise program with
the intention of quitting. Yet, 40 percent of new exercisers don't make it
past the first 3 months.[50] What happened to them? Many inadvertently
exhausted their joy for exercising. Exercising became a chore or a bore,
and no one has time for that. I see you nodding, but it doesn't have to
be that way.

A personal trainer can help, though it's not feasible for most people.
Fortunately, there is another way with no extra cost or fancy equipment
required. Only a matter of mind. And right now, your mind may be too
focused on the goal, and that's a problem.

"Isn't it good to have goals?" you ask, confused.

Absolutely! Goals motivate us to get up off the couch. However, focusing too much on the destination takes away from your experience of the
journey and makes it harder for you to get to the end. Let me illustrate
with this study. Two girlfriends, Gina and Elise, head to the gym for a
workout. Just before hopping on the treadmill, the two are approached
by a researcher who invites them to participate in a study and randomly
assigns them to one of two groups:[51]

Gina is assigned to the **goal group**.

"What is your workout goal?" the researcher asks.

"To lose weight," Gina replies, and she's instructed to focus on her goal
during her workout.

Then the researcher asks, "How long do you plan to run today?"

"Forty-five minutes," Gina replies and hops on the treadmill.

Thirty minutes later, she hops off.

"I'm feeling *terrible* today!" Gina confesses. Gina exercised 15 minutes *less* than she intended.

Elise is assigned to the **experience group**.

"What is your workout experience?" the researcher asks.

"First I stretch and then I run on the treadmill," Elise replies, and she's instructed to focus on her experience during the workout.

Then the researcher asks, "How long do you plan to run today?"

"Thirty-five minutes," Elise replies and hops on the treadmill.

Forty minutes later, she hops off.

"I'm feeling *great* today!" Elise exclaims. Elise exercised 5 minutes *more* than she intended.

For the next 6 weeks, the women continue to work out together.[52] Gina stays focused on her goal and misses nearly a quarter of her workouts. Elise stays focused on her experience and misses only one. By the end of those 6 weeks, Gina *loathes* exercising while Elise is still loving it.

~~The friends continue exercising this way for the next 6 months.~~ Nope: Elise continues exercising this way for the next 6 months. Gina had been spending less and less time at the gym and skipped out on more than half of their planned sessions together. Eventually, Gina quit. What happened to Gina? She was so focused on the destination that she forgot to enjoy the experience, and this made it harder for her to stick with it to the end.

I would have never guessed that a goal mindset could be so detrimental, but it's true and here's why: Exercising is physically challenging. It alters your *inner* world, and this is vacation mode's domain. In contrast, a goal is **extrinsically motivating**. It concerns the *outer* world, and this is work mode's domain. But there is tension between work mode and vacation mode because their objectives are in opposition, and switching back and forth between the two is mentally exhausting.

If only Gina had focused on her experience during exercise, this would have made the whole process more **intrinsically motivating**.[53] What's more, when we focus on our experience during exercise, it becomes **flow-like** — an enjoyable, effortless experience that makes you want to see it through to the end. I can only guess that this is what Arthur Ashe was referring to when he said, "Success is a journey, not a destination. The doing is often more important than the outcome."

The thing I really like about this approach to exercising is that the experience doesn't need to be overly positive to have a positive effect. Focusing on something as neutral as heart rate, heel drive, or glute squeeze will do the trick so long as the focus is here and now.

Still confused about what to do with your goals? Keep 'em! You can have the best of both worlds. Focus on your experience when exercising. Focus on your goals when you are not.

When the Going Gets Tough, the Tough Get Going

Now that you know how to enjoy the journey, it will be easier for you to persevere, especially when the going is *easy*. However, it will still be hard to persevere when the going gets tough. This is when you need your "why," which is about passion and purpose. It helps if your "why" is bigger than you.

Cancer robbed Terry Fox of his leg but spared his life. To him, this was the most incredible gift, and he wanted to give it to others. His goal was to raise $1 million to help fight cancer and prove that a man without a leg was no less a man but maybe even more. He called it the Marathon of Hope. But it wasn't just one marathon; it was nearly 143 marathons that he ran in 143 days as he worked his way across Canada.

He spoke humbly when asked about his incredible accomplishment: "Even though it was so difficult, there was not another thing in the world I would have rather been doing." That's because he wasn't doing it for himself. He was doing it for the kids back at the hospital who were still sick with cancer.

Although Terry Fox is no longer with us, the greatness of his gesture lives on. Every year, people all over Canada run together in his name at the annual Terry Fox Run. It's a highlight of the school year. In the weeks leading up to the event, teachers challenge their students to "Be like Terry." I asked my daughter what that meant to her.

She replied, "To be active . . . and have perseverance."

I read to her what I wrote about Terry, and she reminded me that there was a young boy about her age who had cancer and biked alongside Terry for part of his run. His name was Greg Scott. He had also lost his leg to cancer, and it was too hard for him to run so he pedaled behind. Terry wrote about Greg in his journal: "Greg rode his bike behind me for about 6 miles and it has to be the most inspirational moment I have had!"

Let us never forget that inspiration comes in many different shapes and sizes. So too does greatness.

HOW FOCUS AND CREATIVITY
HELPED ME STICK WITH IT TO THE END

My exercise training had helped me endure one of the most challenging transitions in my life. My goal of completing a full Ironman, something I never thought would be possible, was now well within reach. I had my eyes on the prize, yes, but I was still very much enjoying the process. It was March 2020, and I had almost made it. With my race set for August (only 5 months away, yay!), I could see the light at the end of the tunnel.

Then, the global pandemic canceled the world. Gyms, pools, schools — all closed. Races likely canceled too. How long would we have to live like this? No one knew, and the uncertainty was maddening.

I could feel the tension building in my body. The stress of the situation made it almost impossible for me to train. At times, I wanted to quit but knew that it would do my brain more harm than good. Based on our research, I knew I could continue to train but at a lower intensity. It was a modification I needed for my mental health (see Chapter 3).

Then it occurred to me that other people may not know this. They may be trying to stay well and be healthy, but they may be inadvertently making themselves feel worse. My lab and I wanted to help. We wrote a series of op-eds on how to exercise for mental health. We conducted a survey to gauge how the pandemic was impacting people.[54] Over 1,600 people responded, and the results were devastating. The pandemic was making people anxious, depressed, and distracted. People wanted to exercise to improve their mental health, but stress and anxiety were getting in the way. Those who managed to stay active were coping better. So, we created a toolkit to help others stay active too. You can download the toolkit for free at neurofitlab.com.

I continued to train, but I also struggled to stay focused. Then my race was officially canceled. Now what? And more to the point, how was I going to end this book? There was no indication of when the next official race would be. I couldn't end it with: "They canceled the race, so I didn't do it. The end." Not exactly the inspiring ending I was going for.

Could I train and then complete a full Ironman on my own? Was that even possible? Maybe I could take a page out of Terry's book? Do the Ironman solo and raise money for mental health. Same goal, but with a bigger purpose to help motivate me through to the end.

A Race to the End

The day had finally arrived.

My solo Ironman. (You with me, Terry?)

Ready. Set. Go. The battle was tough. It was hard to endure. But I dug deep.

Why? Because of you. I know it's cheesy, but it's true.

I wanted to show you what it's all about.

A big finale to celebrate the gifts that exercise gives.

Not just for the body. But for the mind too.

Exercise is medicine.

It's the medicine I need.

What's my exercise Rx?

Maybe an Ironman. Maybe not.

What's your exercise Rx?

Any step you choose.

One small step for you, one giant leap for your mental health.

In the end, it's less about the specific exercise prescription and more about the movement.

After moving for 13 hours and 10 minutes straight, I was ready to finish strong. I sprinted across the finish line of the marathon journey that saved my life.

The end.

P.S. I think it's time for me to start a new exercise program. Something less intensive.

Will you join me?

The Achiever Workout

REFERENCE: Chapter 7
MINDSET: Focused and creative

NEURO FIX: Energize and engage
the brain's networks
LEVEL: Advanced

MON	TUES	WED	THURS	FRI	SAT	SUN
Wellness Run	Tenacious Lift	HIIT for Grit	The Neuro Fix	Go Team Go!	Accelerator	

WELLNESS WALK-TO-RUN

Warm up with a 5-minute Wellness Walk. Run for 20 minutes at a comfortably challenging pace. Pay attention to your breath. Cool down with a 5-minute Wellness Walk.

Ready to take the next step? Run 5 minutes longer every week.

TENACIOUS LIFT

Warm up with a 5-minute Wellness Walk, then complete exercises 1 to 5 in Circuit #1 for the prescribed repetitions. Take a 30-second mindful break. Focus on your breathing. Repeat. Then move on to Circuit #2. Repeat.

Circuit #1

ORDER	EXERCISE	REPETITIONS	PICTURED
1	Front Plank	30 seconds	Page 175
2	Kneeling Woodchoppers	10 reps per side	Page 181
3	Sumo Squats	10 reps	Page 197
4	Three-Way Leg Raises	10 reps per way	Page 199
5	High Knees	30 seconds	Page 176
	Mindful Break	30 seconds	

Circuit #2

ORDER	EXERCISE	REPETITIONS	PICTURED
1	Bicycles	10 reps per side	Page 169
2	Deadlifts	10 reps	Page 174
3	Pushups	10 reps	Page 185
4	Reverse Flies	10 reps	Page 186
5	Mountain Climbers	30 seconds	Page 184
	Mindful Break	30 seconds	

Ready to take the next step? Increase your repetitions to 15 reps and 40 seconds. Repeat the exercises a third time. *Advanced progressions:* Circuit #1: 1. Front Plank to Single Leg Front Plank, add reaches or do on unstable surface; 2. Add weight; 3. Add weight; 4. Add resistance band. Circuit #2: 2. Add weight; 3. Do on a decline or unstable surface and change the tempo; 4. Add weight.

HIIT FOR GRIT

Warm up for 5 minutes, then HIIT it. Do 1 minute with hard effort followed by 1 minute with easy effort; repeat ten times. Can be done while running, cycling, or stair-climbing, indoors or outdoors. Feel free to mix it up for maximum grit.

Ready to take the next step? Add an incline or resistance to your hard effort.

THE NEURO FIX

(Do it anywhere, anytime you need it): Warm up with a 5-minute Wellness Walk, then complete exercises 1 to 4. Work as hard as you can. Repeat.

ORDER	EXERCISE	REPETITIONS	PICTURED
1	Jumping Jacks	30 seconds	Page 178
2	Mountain Climbers	30 seconds	Page 184
3	Skaters	30 seconds	Page 193
4	High Knees	30 seconds	Page 176

THE ACCELERATOR

Warm up with a 5-minute Wellness Walk, then complete exercises 1 to 5 in Circuit #1 for the prescribed repetitions. Take a 30-second mindful break. Focus on your breathing. Repeat. Then move on to Circuit #2. Repeat.

Circuit #1

ORDER	EXERCISE	REPETITIONS	PICTURED
1	Dead Bugs	10 reps per side	Page 173
2	Side Plank	30 seconds	Page 190
3	Squats	10 reps	Page 195
4	Supine Hip Lifts	10 reps	Page 198
5	Skaters	30 seconds	Page 193
	Mindful Break	30 seconds	

Circuit #2

ORDER	EXERCISE	REPETITIONS	PICTURED
1	V Sit	30 seconds	Page 200
2	Split Squats	10 reps per side	Page 194
3	Row	10 reps	Page 187
4	Shoulder Presses	10 reps	Page 188
5	Jumping Jacks	30 seconds	Page 178
	Mindful Break	30 seconds	

Ready to take the next step? Increase your repetitions to 15 reps and 40 seconds. Repeat the exercises a third time. *Advanced progressions*: Circuit #1: 2. Do on unstable surface; 3. Add weight; 4. Add weight, marches, or do with single leg. Circuit #2: 1. Arms raised overhead; Add weight to workouts 2 to 4.

GO TEAM GO!

Play your favorite sport. Have fun!

ACKNOWLEDGMENTS

I would like to thank the team at HarperCollins for helping me translate the science and stories into a real book, including my editor Karen Murgolo and her assistant Jacqueline Quirk; Melissa Lotfy and Chloe Foster for art direction; Marina Padakis and Christina Stambaugh in managing editorial; Bridget Nocera in publicity; and Katie Tull in marketing. I would like to thank my agent Chris Bucci of Aevitas Creative Management for championing my ideas and supporting me through the entire process.

Thanks to my colleagues in the field and my incredible research team in the NeuroFit Lab for generating such incredible evidence for the benefits of exercise on the brain, and to my former graduate student, Alexis Bullock, for helping me fact check all the notes.

I would like to acknowledge my coach Kristina Plachecki, aka Coach K (placheckicoaching.ca), for helping to design the evidence-informed exercise programs included at the end of each chapter. I would also like to acknowledge photographer Paulina Rzeczkowska (www.paulinarz.com) for beautifully capturing my family, friends, and me demonstrating those exercises for you at the back of the book.

A huge shout-out to my family, friends, students, and colleagues for your enduring support, and to my darling daughter Monica for all of your inspiration.

APPENDIX: EXERCISES

> **Note:** No weights? No problem. You can substitute weighted household items like cans, laundry detergent, or rocks in a bag or anything with a handle.

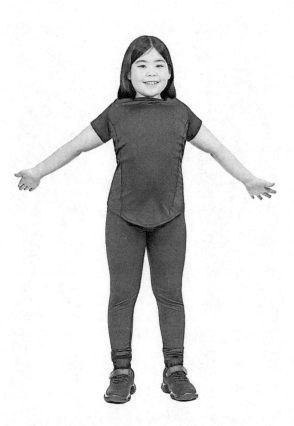

Arm Circles (backward): Stand tall with your feet shoulder-width apart and arms by your sides. Straighten and extend each arm. Rotate each arm backward to make a circle. Move arms in synchrony.

Arm Circles (forward): Stand tall with your feet shoulder-width apart and arms by your sides. Straighten and extend each arm. Rotate each arm forward to make a circle. Move arms in synchrony.

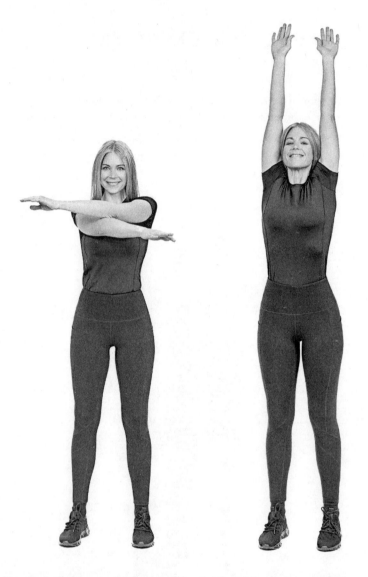

Arm Swings (across the body): Stand tall with your feet shoulder-width apart. Straighten and extend your arms out in front of you at shoulder height. Hold this position while you open your arms away from each other and then bring them back together, crossing them in front.

Arm Swings (up and down): Stand tall with your feet shoulder-width apart and arms by your sides. Straighten and extend your arms up overhead. Reach for the sky. Then bring them back down to your sides.

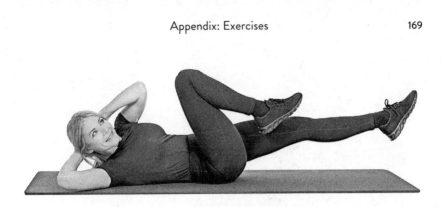

Bicycles: Lie down on your back with your hands behind your head and knees bent with shins parallel to the ceiling. Engage your core and lift your chest off the ground as you bring your left elbow toward your right knee while extending your left leg out in front of you. Lower yourself back to the starting position and then switch sides.

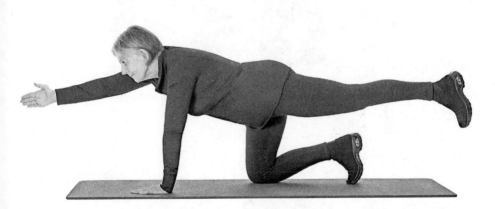

Bird Dogs: Get on your hands and knees with your hands directly underneath your shoulders and your knees directly underneath your hips. Engage your core. Stretch and reach your right arm and left leg away from your body. Keep right thumb pointed up toward the ceiling. Bring your arm and leg back to the starting position and then switch sides. Keep your hips level throughout the movement. *Bird Dog Holds* involve the same movement, but you hold your arm and leg up and away from your body for the prescribed duration and then switch sides.

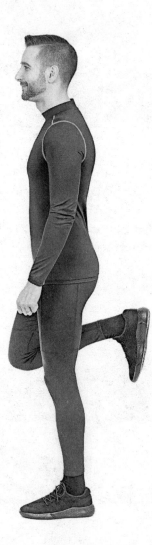

Butt Kicks: Stand tall with your feet shoulder-width apart, knees slightly bent, and your arms by your side. Kick your right foot back toward your right glute and then return to starting position. Repeat with your left foot.

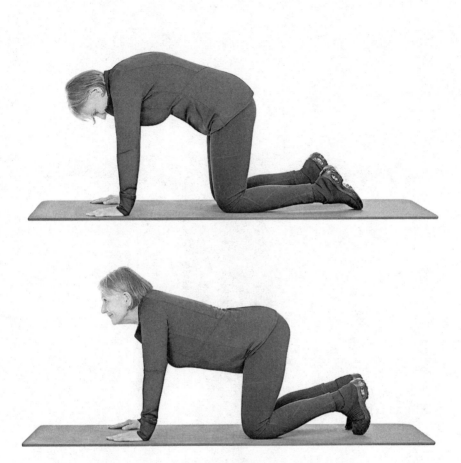

Cat Cow: Get on your hands and knees with your hands directly underneath your shoulders and your knees directly underneath your hips. Engage your core. For cat pose, tuck your tailbone in while you arch your upper back and tuck your head with eyes looking at knees. For cow pose, tilt your tailbone back while pushing your shoulder blades back and lifting your head with eyes forward. Alternate between cat and cow poses.

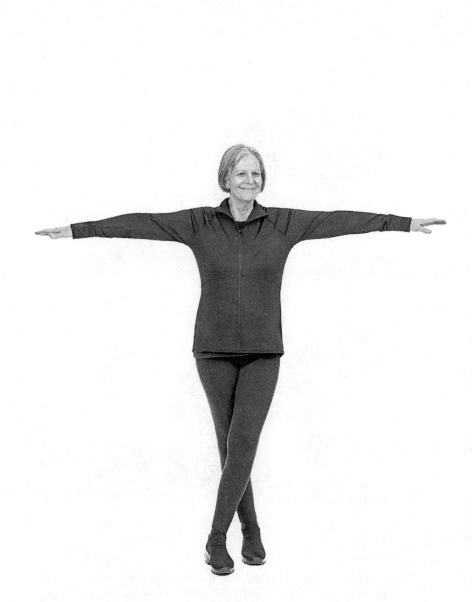

Crossovers: Stand tall with your feet shoulder-width apart and your arms outstretched. Step to the right with your right foot. Swing your left foot behind your right foot and then in front of it, touching down with your toe for balance when needed. End the sequence by stepping your left foot back to the starting position. Complete all reps before switching sides.

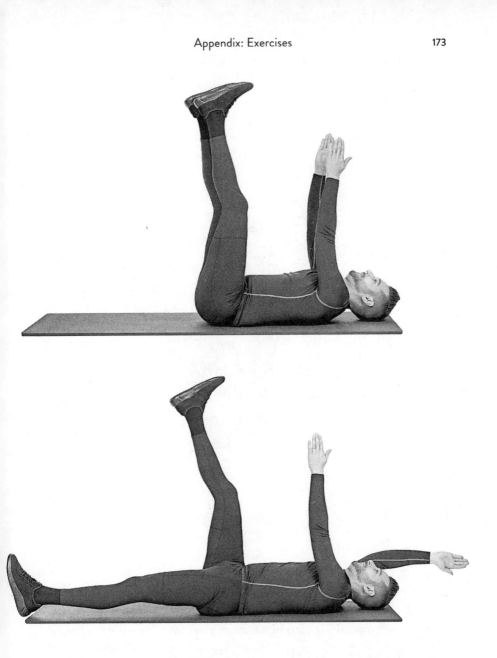

Dead Bugs: Lie on your back. Point your arms and legs straight up in the air, positioning your arms over shoulders and your legs over hips. Engage your core. Slowly extend and lower your right arm backward (behind your head) and your left leg forward (in front of your body). Stop just before your arm touches the ground. Now, bring that arm and leg back to their starting positions. Repeat the movement with your left arm and right leg.

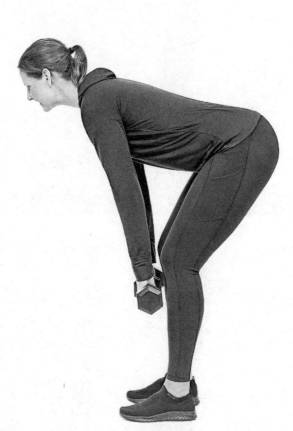

Deadlifts: Stand tall with your feet shoulder-width apart and arms in front of you with a weight in each hand and palms facing your body. Engage your core. Bring your hips back as you lower the weights in front of your body to the tops of your shins. Keep your back flat and knees slightly bent. Bring your hips forward and straighten your legs to return to the starting position. Keep your arms straight and your shoulders strong throughout the movement.

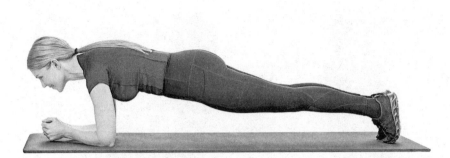

Front Plank: Lie down facing the ground. Lift your body up with your forearms (elbows underneath your shoulders) and toes (so that your back is parallel to the ground). Hold this position while engaging your core. *Single Leg Front Plank* involves the same position but with one leg lifted. Hold this position while engaging your core. Switch legs and repeat.

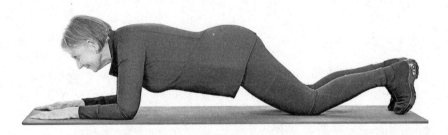

Front Plank (modified): Lie down facing the ground. Lift your body up with your forearms (elbows underneath your shoulders) and position knees on the ground so that your back is parallel to the ground. Hold this position while engaging your core.

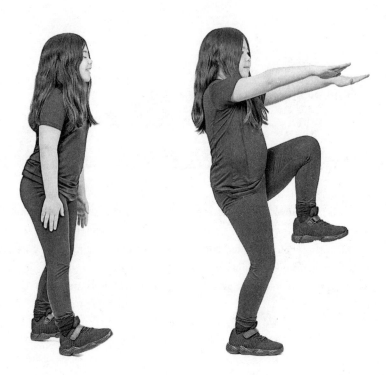

Heel Walk: Stand tall with your feet shoulder-width apart and your arms in a comfortable position. Walk forward on your heels.

High Knees: Stand tall with your feet shoulder-width apart. Arms stretched out in front of you. While running in place, lift knees up high to your waist, keeping your body tall and feet flexed toward your shins.

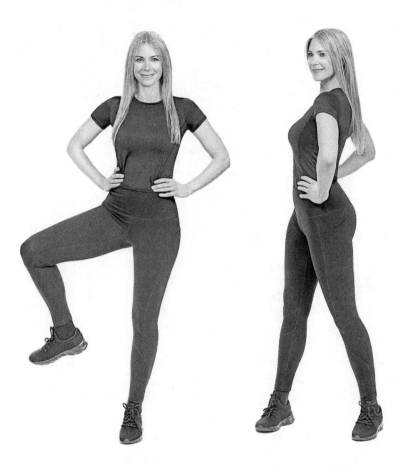

Hip Openers: Stand tall with your feet shoulder-width apart and your arms in a comfortable position. Raise your right knee up and out in front of your body to hip height and rotate it to the right side of your body. Touch down your right foot behind your body. Then raise it up again to hip height before rotating it back to the starting position. Complete all reps before switching sides.

Hip Twists: Stand tall with your feet shoulder-width apart and your hands on your hips. Keep your lower body facing forward, engage your core, and rotate your upper body to the right and then to the left. Move in a slow and controlled manner.

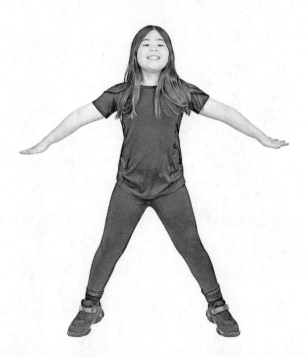

Jumping Jacks: Stand tall with your feet shoulder-width apart. Jump up, kicking both feet out while you extend your arms up overhead toward each other. On your way back down, return your legs together and arms to your sides.

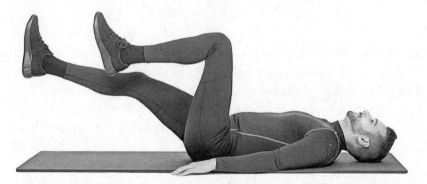

Kickouts: Lie on your back with arms by your side. Bend your hips and knees so that knees are directly above your hips with shins parallel to the ground. Engage your core. Slowly extend your right leg while keeping your back flat. Bring your right leg back to the starting position. Repeat the movement with your left leg.

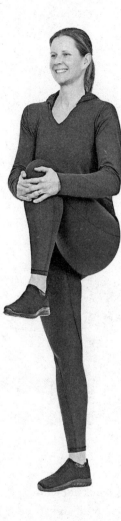

Knee Tucks: Stand tall with your feet shoulder-width apart. Bend your left leg to your waist, grab it with both hands, and give it a tug. Then lower. Repeat with your right leg.

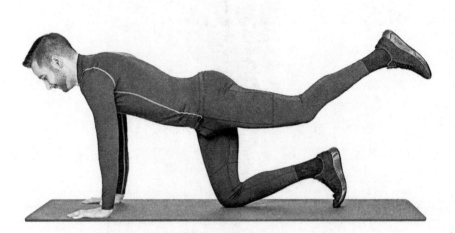

Kneeling Donkey Kicks: Get on your hands and knees with your hands directly underneath your shoulders and your knees directly underneath your hips. Engage your core. Extend and lift your left leg out behind you and then bring it back to the starting position. Keep hips level throughout the movement. Complete all the repetitions for one leg and then switch legs.

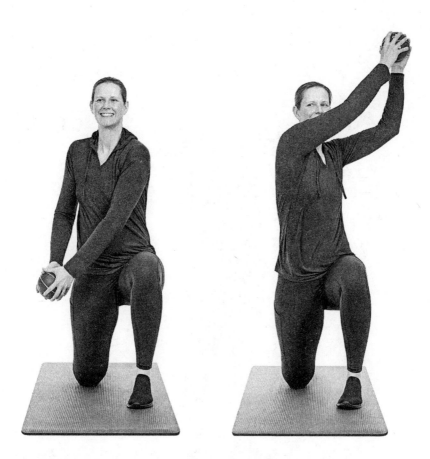

Kneeling Woodchoppers: Get down on your right knee. Position your left leg forward with knee bent at a 90-degree angle and foot flat on the ground. Engage your core and hold a weight with both hands. Extend your arms as you move the weight diagonally across your body from below your right hip to above your left shoulder. Complete all reps for one side. Switch leg positions and repeat.

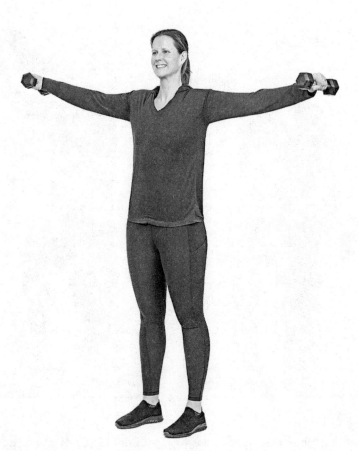

Lateral Raises: Stand tall with your feet about shoulder-width apart, arms by your sides, holding dumbbells with palms facing your body. Lift the weights by extending your arms straight out from the side of your body up until you reach shoulder height and then lower back down. Keep your elbows soft throughout the movement. This movement can also be performed in a *bent-over* position with upper body parallel to the floor.

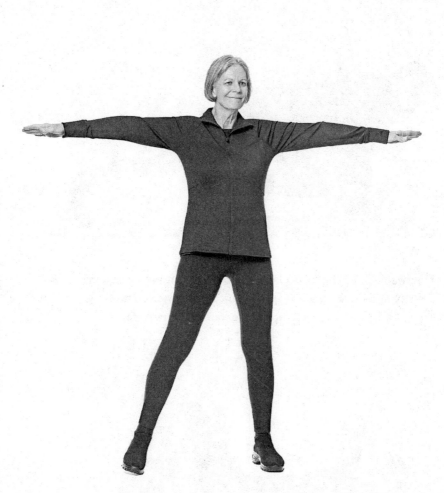

Lateral Step Gathers: Stand tall with your feet shoulder-width apart and your arms outstretched. Step to the right with your right foot and bring your left foot to meet it. Then, step to the left with your left foot and bring your right foot to meet it.

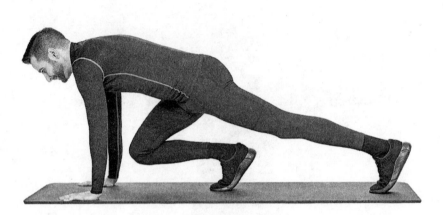

Mountain Climbers: Do a plank. Bend your right knee and bring it directly under your body as far as you can. Then as you return your right leg to its starting position, repeat the movement with your left leg.

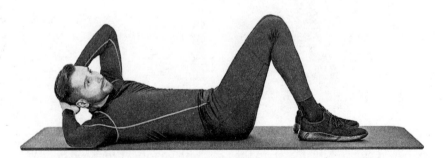

Oblique Twists: Lie down on your back with your hands behind your head and your knees bent with feet flat on the ground. Engage your core and lift your chest off the ground as you bring your left elbow toward your right knee. Keep your lower body still. Return to the starting position and switch sides.

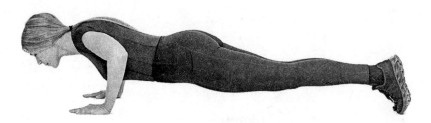

Pushups: Lie facing the ground with your hands and toes on the ground. The rest of your body should be off the ground. Your hands should be greater than shoulder-width apart with your elbows in line with your chest. Your toes should be far enough away from your hands so that your whole body is in a straight line. Lower your body as far as you can without touching the ground and then push yourself back up to the starting position.

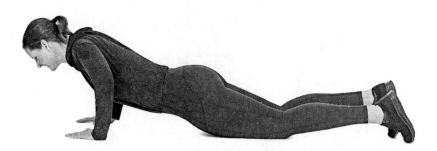

Pushups (modified): Get down on your hands and knees. Your hands should be greater than shoulder-width apart with your elbows in line with your chest. Your knees should be far enough away from your hands so that there is a straight line from your knees to your shoulders. Lower your body as far as you can without touching the ground and then push yourself back up to the starting position. Modified pushups can also be done against a *wall*. Stand an arm's length away from the wall with your back straight, hips square, and hands on wall. Bend your elbows and lean into the wall as far as you can without touching it and then push yourself back to the starting position.

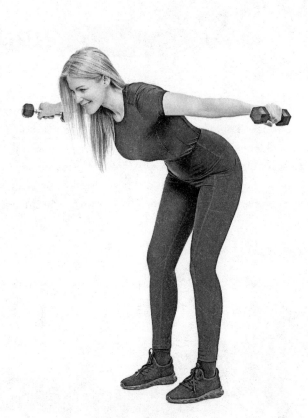

Reverse Flies: Bend forward with knees slightly bent, back straight, and chest facing the ground at a 45-degree angle. With straight arms positioned underneath your chest, hold a dumbbell in each hand with palms facing each other. Lift the weights away from each other to shoulder height, making a "T," and then lower to starting position.

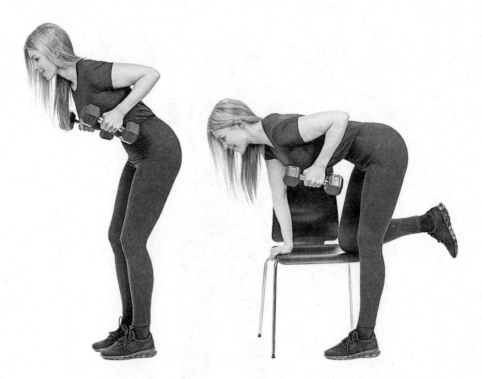

Row: Bend forward with knees slightly bent, back straight, and chest facing the ground at a 45-degree angle. With straight arms positioned underneath your chest, hold a dumbbell in each hand with palms facing each other. Keeping your elbows close to your body, bend your elbows back to lift the weights behind your body. Then return to starting position. The same movement can be performed one arm at a time (i.e., *single arm*). Complete all reps for one arm before switching sides.

Row (supported): Bend forward with knees slightly bent, back straight, and chest facing the ground. Support yourself by holding on or kneeling on a sturdy support like a chair or bench. With your other arm straight and positioned underneath your chest, hold a dumbbell in your hand with palm facing you. Keeping your elbows close to your body, bend your elbow back to lift the weight behind your body. Then return to starting position. Complete all reps for one arm before switching sides.

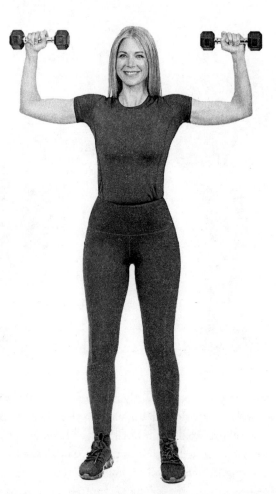

Shoulder Presses: Stand tall with your feet about shoulder-width apart and a dumbbell in each hand. Bend your elbows and lift them to shoulder height. Start with the dumbbells in line with the bottom of your ears, palms facing forward. Extend your arms up, bring the dumbbells together overhead, and then return to starting position. Add a *Bicep Curl* by starting with the dumbbells by your sides, palms facing forward. Curl the dumbbells up toward your shoulders, twist your wrists so your palms are facing forward, and extend your arms up to execute the shoulder press. Return to the starting position by first lowering the dumbbells to your shoulders, twisting your wrists so your palms are facing you, and lowering to starting position.

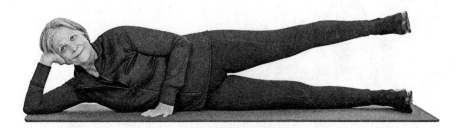

Side-Lying Hip Abduction: Lie down on your side so that your hips are stacked on top of each other and your head is supported by your arm or hand. Engage your core. Keeping your top leg straight and foot flexed, lift it up until it's just past your shoulder while positioning your top foot parallel to the ground. Lower it back down until it's just above the bottom leg. Complete all reps before switching sides.

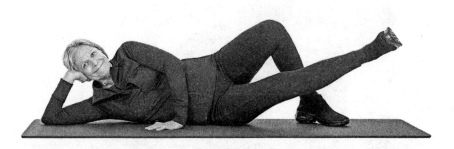

Side-Lying Hip Adduction: Lie down on left side so that your hips are stacked on top of each other and your head is supported by your arm or hand. Engage your core and place your right arm in front of you for support. Bend your right leg and place it behind your left knee so that your right foot is firmly planted on the ground. Now, keeping your left leg straight and foot flexed, lift it up toward shoulder level while positioning your foot parallel to the ground. Lower it back down until it's just above the ground. Complete all reps before switching sides.

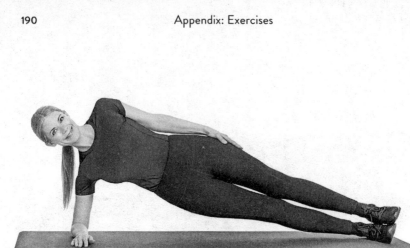

Side Plank: Lie down on your left side with feet stacked on top of each other. Lift your body up with your bottom forearm (elbow underneath your shoulder) and feet (so that your back is flat). Hold this position while engaging your core. Hold for the prescribed duration before switching sides.

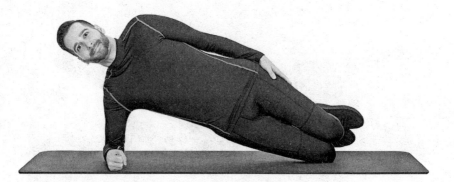

Side Plank (modified): Lie down on your left side with knees bent and feet and knees stacked. Lift your body up with your bottom forearm (elbow underneath your shoulder) and knee (past your hips so that your back is flat). Hold this position while engaging your core. Hold for the prescribed duration before switching sides.

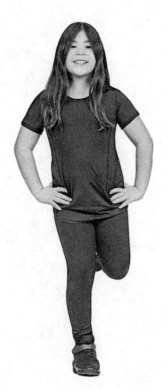

Single-Leg Balance: Stand tall with your hands on your hips and slowly lift one leg off the ground while balancing on the other. Keep your core engaged and hips level. Close your eyes for added difficulty. Repeat with other leg.

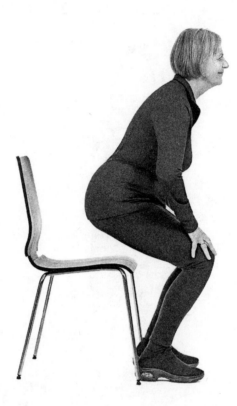

Sit Stands: Sit tall on a chair with your feet shoulder-width apart and your arms by your sides or resting on your knees. Without leaning forward, press off with your feet and stand up tall. Sit back down with control.

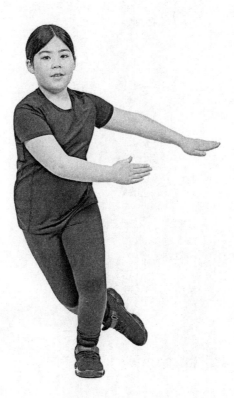

Skaters: Stand tall with your feet shoulder-width apart. Bend your knees. Hop to the left with your left foot while you transfer your body weight to your left leg and bring your right foot behind your left foot, just past it, and not touching the ground. Push off from your left foot and hop to the right with your right foot as you transfer your body weight to your right leg and swing your left foot behind your right foot without touching the ground.

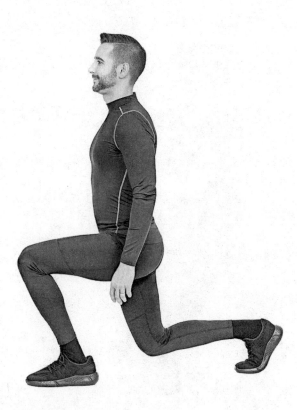

Split Squats: Stand with your feet about shoulder-width apart and with one foot about 3 feet in front of the other. While leaning forward slightly from the waist, lower your body down to the ground while bending your knees so that your front foot remains flat and your back foot is on its toes. Then press into the ground with your feet and stand back up to the starting position. Switch the front and back leg once all of the repetitions have been completed.

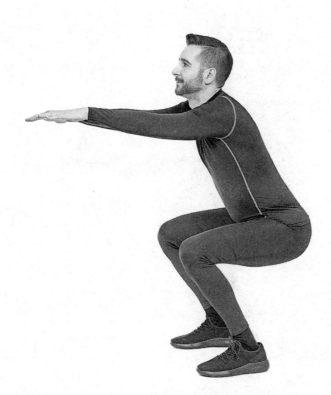

Squats: Stand tall with your feet about shoulder-width apart and your arms stretched out in front of you. As if you were going to sit in a chair, bend your knees and lower your body down while keeping your chest up. Lower down as much as you can with control and then press into the ground with your feet and stand back up. For a *supported squat*, hold a sturdy support like a chair or countertop while performing the squat.

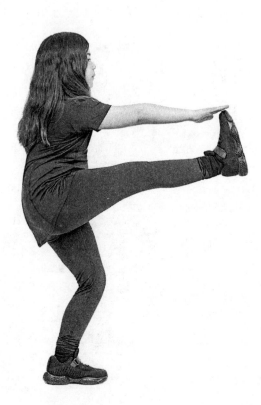

Straight-Leg Kicks: Stand tall with your feet shoulder-width apart. Stretch out your right arm in front of you at shoulder height. Kick up your right leg in front of your body, keeping your leg straight and body tall. Repeat with your left arm and leg.

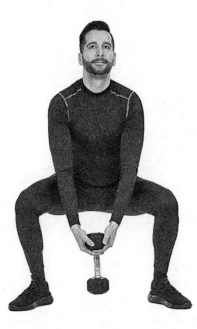

Sumo Squats: Stand tall with your feet wider than shoulder-width and your toes pointed out to the side. Hold the top of a dumbbell in front of you below your waist with your arms fully extended. As if you were going to sit in a chair, bend your knees and lower your body down while keeping your chest up. Lower down as much as you can with control and then press into the ground with your feet and stand back up.

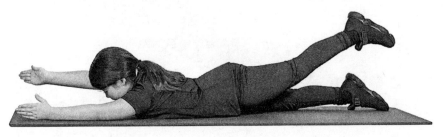

Superman (alternating): Lie on your stomach with legs and arms fully extended, thumbs up and toes pointed. Engage your core and gently lift and extend your right arm and left leg and then bring them back down to the ground. Repeat the same movement with your left arm and right leg. Alternate between sides for the prescribed repetitions. *Superman* involves the same movement, but you raise both arms and legs at the same time and hold for the prescribed duration.

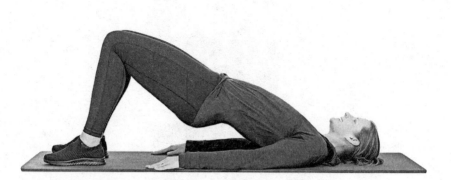

Supine Hip Hold: Lie on your back with your arms by your side and your legs bent and hip-width apart. Make sure that your feet are flat on the ground past your knees and away from your body. Push into the ground with your feet to lift your hips. Keep your body flat from your knees to your shoulders and hold.

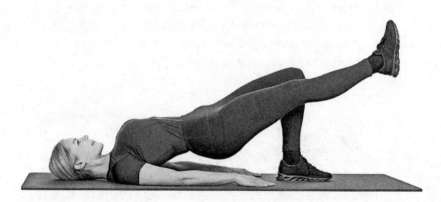

Supine Hip Lifts: Same as Supine Hip Hold but instead of holding, lift and lower your hips. For the *single-leg* modification, instead of placing two feet flat on the ground, place only one foot on the ground at a time. Keep your other leg straight and hovering above the ground. Complete all reps before switching sides.

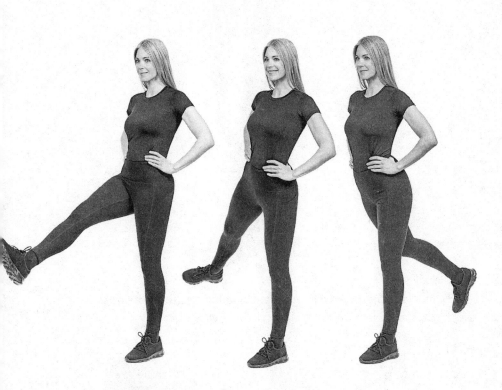

Three-Way Leg Raises: Stand tall with your feet hip-width apart and core engaged. Lift your right leg out in front of your body and back to the starting position. Now lift that same leg out to the side of your body and back to the starting position. And finally, lift that same leg directly behind you (don't lean forward) and back to the starting position. Keep your leg straight and foot flexed through the entire movement. Complete all the repetitions on one side before switching sides.

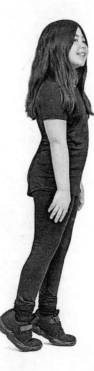

Toe Walk: Stand tall with your feet shoulder-width apart and your arms in a comfortable position. Walk forward on your toes.

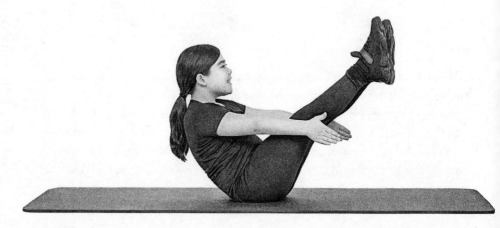

V Sit: Sit down on the ground. Lean back onto your tailbone. Lift your legs off the ground while keeping your back and legs straight. Stretch your arms out in front of you. Hold this position for the prescribed amount of time.

REFERENCES

1. The Reasons It's Hard to Exercise

1. Blundell, J., Gibbons, C., Caudwell, P., Finlayson, G. & Hopkins, M. Appetite control and energy balance: Impact of exercise. *Obesity Reviews* **16**, 67–76 (2015).

2. Liebenberg, L. Persistence hunting by modern hunter-gatherers. *Current Anthropology* **47**, 1017–1026 (2006).

3. Selinger, J.C., O'Connor, S.M., Wong, J.D. & Donelan, J.M. Humans can continuously optimize energetic cost during walking. *Current Biology* **25**, 2452–2456 (2015).

4. Englert, C. & Rummel, J. I want to keep on exercising but I don't: The negative impact of momentary lacks of self-control on exercise adherence. *Psychology of Sport and Exercise* **26**, 24–31 (2016).

5. Harris, S. & Bray, S.R. Effects of mental fatigue on exercise decision-making. *Psychology of Sport and Exercise* **44**, 1–8 (2019).

6. Cheval, B., *et al.* Avoiding sedentary behaviors requires more cortical resources than avoiding physical activity: An EEG study. *Neuropsychologia* **119**, 68–80 (2018).

7. Arbour, K.P. & Martin Ginis, K.A. A randomised controlled trial of the effects of implementation intentions on women's walking behaviour. *Psychology and Health* **24**, 49–65 (2009).

8. Reed, J.L. & Pipe, A.L. The talk test: A useful tool for prescribing and monitoring exercise intensity. *Current Opinion in Cardiology* **29**, 475–480 (2014).

9. Williamson, J., McColl, R., Mathews, D., Ginsburg, M. & Mitchell, J. Activation of the insular cortex is affected by the intensity of exercise. *Journal of Applied Physiology* **87**, 1213–1219 (1999).

10. Scherr, J., *et al.* Associations between Borg's rating of perceived exertion

and physiological measures of exercise intensity. *European Journal of Applied Physiology* **113**, 147–155 (2013).

11. Parfitt, G., Rose, E.A. & Burgess, W.M. The psychological and physiological responses of sedentary individuals to prescribed and preferred intensity exercise. *British Journal of Health Psychology* **11**, 39–53 (2006).

12. Hardy, C.J. & Rejeski, W.J. Not what, but how one feels: The measurement of affect during exercise. *Journal of Sport and Exercise Psychology* **11**, 304–317 (1989).

13. Borg, G.A. Psychophysical bases of perceived exertion. *Medicine & Science in Sports & Exercise* (1982).

14. Messonnier, L.A., *et al.* Lactate kinetics at the lactate threshold in trained and untrained men. *Journal of Applied Physiology* **114**, 1593–1602 (2013).

15. Ekkekakis, P., Hall, E.E. & Petruzzello, S.J. The relationship between exercise intensity and affective responses demystified: To crack the 40-year-old nut, replace the 40-year-old nutcracker! *Annals of Behavioral Medicine* **35**, 136–149 (2008).

16. Acevedo, E., Kraemer, R., Haltom, R. & Tryniecki, J. Perceptual responses proximal to the onset. *Journal of Sports Medicine & Physical Fitness* **43**, 267–273 (2003).

17. Williams, D.M., *et al.* Acute affective response to a moderate-intensity exercise stimulus predicts physical activity participation 6 and 12 months later. *Psychology of Sport and Exercise* **9**, 231–245 (2008).

18. Seiler, S. What is best practice for training intensity and duration distribution in endurance athletes? *International Journal of Sports Physiology and Performance* **5**, 276–291 (2010).

19. Bargai, N., Ben-Shakhar, G. & Shalev, A.Y. Posttraumatic stress disorder and depression in battered women: The mediating role of learned helplessness. *Journal of Family Violence* **22**, 267–275 (2007).

20. Maier, S.F. & Seligman, M.E. Learned helplessness at fifty: Insights from neuroscience. *Psychological Review* **123**, 349 (2016).

21. Silverman, M.N. & Deuster, P.A. Biological mechanisms underlying the role of physical fitness in health and resilience. *Interface Focus* **4**, 20140040 (2014).

22. Greenwood, B.N. & Fleshner, M. Exercise, stress resistance, and central serotonergic systems. *Exercise and Sport Sciences Reviews* **39**, 140 (2011).

23. Rimmele, U., *et al.* Trained men show lower cortisol, heart rate and psychological responses to psychosocial stress compared with untrained men. *Psychoneuroendocrinology* **32**, 627–635 (2007).

24. von Haaren, B., Haertel, S., Stumpp, J., Hey, S. & Ebner-Priemer, U. Reduced emotional stress reactivity to a real-life academic examination stressor in students participating in a 20-week aerobic exercise training: A randomised controlled trial using Ambulatory Assessment. *Psychology of Sport and Exercise* **20**, 67–75 (2015).

25. Silverman, M.N. & Deuster, P.A. Biological mechanisms underlying the role of physical fitness in health and resilience. *Interface Focus* **4**, 20140040 (2014).

26. Kitraki, E., Karandrea, D. & Kittas, C. Long-lasting effects of stress on glucocorticoid receptor gene expression in the rat brain. *Neuroendocrinology* **69**, 331–338 (1999).

27. Labonte, B., *et al.* Differential glucocorticoid receptor exon 1B, 1C, and 1H expression and methylation in suicide completers with a history of childhood abuse. *Biological Psychiatry* **72**, 41–48 (2012).

28. Cohen, S., *et al.* Chronic stress, glucocorticoid receptor resistance, inflammation, and disease risk. *Proceedings of the National Academy of Sciences* **109**, 5995–5999 (2012).

29. Lupien, S.J., McEwen, B.S., Gunnar, M.R. & Heim, C. Effects of stress throughout the lifespan on the brain, behaviour and cognition. *Nature Reviews Neuroscience* **10**, 434–445 (2009).

30. Adlard, P. & Cotman, C. Voluntary exercise protects against stress-induced decreases in brain-derived neurotrophic factor protein expression. *Neuroscience* **124**, 985–992 (2004).

31. Marais, L., Stein, D.J. & Daniels, W.M. Exercise increases BDNF levels in the striatum and decreases depressive-like behavior in chronically stressed rats. *Metabolic Brain Disease* **24**, 587–597 (2009).

32. Zschucke, E., Renneberg, B., Dimeo, F., Wüstenberg, T. & Ströhle, A. The stress-buffering effect of acute exercise: Evidence for HPA axis negative feedback. *Psychoneuroendocrinology* **51**, 414–425 (2015).

33. Stults-Kolehmainen, M.A., Bartholomew, J.B. & Sinha, R. Chronic psychological stress impairs recovery of muscular function and somatic sensations over a 96-hour period. *The Journal of Strength & Conditioning Research* **28**, 2007–2017 (2014).

34. Perna, F.M. & McDowell, S.L. Role of psychological stress in cortisol recovery from exhaustive exercise among elite athletes. *International Journal of Behavioral Medicine* **2**, 13 (1995).

35. Lucibello, K.M., Paolucci, E.M., Graham, J.D. & Heisz, J.J. A randomized control trial investigating high-intensity interval training and mental health: A novel non-responder phenotype related to anxiety in young adults. *Mental Health and Physical Activity*, **18**, 100327 (2020).

36. Soya, H., *et al.* BDNF induction with mild exercise in the rat hippocampus. *Biochemical and Biophysical Research Communications* **358**, 961–967 (2007).

37. Bood, R.J., Nijssen, M., Van Der Kamp, J. & Roerdink, M. The power of auditory-motor synchronization in sports: Enhancing running performance by coupling cadence with the right beats. *PLOS ONE* **8** (2013).

38. De Ataide e Silva, T., *et al.* Can carbohydrate mouth rinse improve performance during exercise? A systematic review. *Nutrients* **6**, 1–10 (2014).

2. Move Away from Anxiety and Pain

1. Bandelow, B. & Michaelis, S. Epidemiology of anxiety disorders in the 21st century. *Dialogues in Clinical Neuroscience* **17**, 327 (2015).
2. Watson, J.B. & Rayner, R. Conditioned emotional reactions. *Journal of Experimental Psychology* **3**, 1 (1920).
3. El Khoury-Malhame, M., *et al.* Amygdala activity correlates with attentional bias in PTSD. *Neuropsychologia* **49**, 1969–1973 (2011).
4. Zhou, Z., *et al.* Genetic variation in human NPY expression affects stress response and emotion. *Nature* **452**, 997–1001 (2008).
5. Zhou, Z., *et al.* Genetic variation in human NPY expression affects stress response and emotion. *Nature* **452**, 997–1001 (2008).
6. Fendt, M., *et al.* Fear-reducing effects of intra-amygdala neuropeptide Y infusion in animal models of conditioned fear: An NPY Y1 receptor independent effect. *Psychopharmacology* **206**, 291–301 (2009).
7. Sah, R., *et al.* Low cerebrospinal fluid neuropeptide Y concentrations in posttraumatic stress disorder. *Biological Psychiatry* **66**, 705–707 (2009).
8. Rämson, R., Jürimäe, J., Jürimäe, T. & Mäestu, J. The effect of 4-week training period on plasma neuropeptide Y, leptin and ghrelin responses in male rowers. *European Journal of Applied Physiology* **112**, 1873–1880 (2012).
9. Lucibello, K., Parker, J. & Heisz, J. Examining a training effect on the state anxiety response to an acute bout of exercise in low and high anxious individuals. *Journal of Affective Disorders* **247**, 29–35 (2019).
10. Stubbs, B., *et al.* An examination of the anxiolytic effects of exercise for people with anxiety and stress-related disorders: A meta-analysis. *Psychiatry Research* **249**, 102–108 (2017).
11. Ensari, I., Greenlee, T.A., Motl, R.W. & Petruzzello, S.J. Meta-analysis of acute exercise effects on state anxiety: An update of randomized controlled trials over the past 25 years. *Depression and Anxiety* **32**, 624–634 (2015).
12. Stubbs, B., *et al.* An examination of the anxiolytic effects of exercise for people with anxiety and stress-related disorders: A meta-analysis. *Psychiatry Research* **249**, 102–108 (2017).
13. Gordon, B.R., McDowell, C.P., Lyons, M. & Herring, M.P. The effects of resistance exercise training on anxiety: A meta-analysis and meta-regression analysis of randomized controlled trials. *Sports Medicine* **47**, 2521–2532 (2017).
14. Cramer, H., *et al.* Yoga for anxiety: A systematic review and meta-analysis of randomized controlled trials. *Depression and Anxiety* **35**, 830–843 (2018).
15. Wang, F., *et al.* The effects of tai chi on depression, anxiety, and psychological well-being: A systematic review and meta-analysis. *International Journal of Behavioral Medicine* **21**, 605–617 (2014).
16. Raeder, F., Merz, C.J., Margraf, J. & Zlomuzica, A. The association between fear extinction, the ability to accomplish exposure and exposure therapy outcome in specific phobia. *Scientific Reports* **10**, 1–11 (2020).

17. Keyan, D. & Bryant, R.A. Acute exercise-induced enhancement of fear inhibition is moderated by BDNF Val66Met polymorphism. *Translational Psychiatry* **9**, 1–10 (2019).
18. Tanner, M.K., Hake, H.S., Bouchet, C.A. & Greenwood, B.N. Running from fear: Exercise modulation of fear extinction. *Neurobiology of Learning and Memory* **151**, 28–34 (2018).
19. Asmundson, G.J., *et al*. Let's get physical: A contemporary review of the anxiolytic effects of exercise for anxiety and its disorders. *Depression and Anxiety* **30**, 362–373 (2013).
20. Smits, J.A., *et al*. Reducing anxiety sensitivity with exercise. *Depression and Anxiety* **25**, 689–699 (2008).
21. Sabourin, B.C., Hilchey, C.A., Lefaivre, M.-J., Watt, M.C. & Stewart, S.H. Why do they exercise less? Barriers to exercise in high-anxiety-sensitive women. *Cognitive Behaviour Therapy* **40**, 206–215 (2011).
22. Moshier, S.J., *et al*. Clarifying the link between distress intolerance and exercise: Elevated anxiety sensitivity predicts less vigorous exercise. *Cognitive Therapy and Research* **37**, 476–482 (2013).
23. Esquivel, G., *et al*. Acute exercise reduces the effects of a 35% CO2 challenge in patients with panic disorder. *Journal of Affective Disorders* **107**, 217–220 (2008).
24. Plag, J., Ergec, D.L., Fydrich, T. & Ströhle, A. High-intensity interval training in panic disorder patients: A pilot study. *The Journal of Nervous and Mental Disease* **207**, 184–187 (2019).
25. Spindler, H. & Pedersen, S.S. Posttraumatic stress disorder in the wake of heart disease: Prevalence, risk factors, and future research directions. *Psychosomatic Medicine* **67**, 715–723 (2005).
26. Edmondson, D., *et al*. Prevalence of PTSD in survivors of stroke and transient ischemic attack: A meta-analytic review. *PLOS ONE* **8**, e66435 (2013).
27. Fang, J., Ayala, C., Luncheon, C., Ritchey, M. & Loustalot, F. Use of outpatient cardiac rehabilitation among heart attack survivors — 20 states and the District of Columbia, 2013 and four states, 2015. *Morbidity and Mortality Weekly Report* **66**, 869 (2017).
28. Ter Hoeve, N., *et al*. Does cardiac rehabilitation after an acute cardiac syndrome lead to changes in physical activity habits? Systematic review. *Physical Therapy* **95**, 167–179 (2015).
29. Farris, S.G., Bond, D.S., Wu, W.C., Stabile, L.M. & Abrantes, A.M. Anxiety sensitivity and fear of exercise in patients attending cardiac rehabilitation. *Mental Health and Physical Activity* **15**, 22–26 (2018).
30. Edmondson, D., *et al*. Posttraumatic stress due to an acute coronary syndrome increases risk of 42-month major adverse cardiac events and all-cause mortality. *Journal of Psychiatric Research* **45**, 1621–1626 (2011).
31. Dahlhamer, J., *et al*. Prevalence of chronic pain and high-impact chronic pain among adults — United States, 2016. *Morbidity and Mortality Weekly Report* **67**, 1001 (2018).

32. Slade, S.C., Patel, S., Underwood, M. & Keating, J.L. What are patient beliefs and perceptions about exercise for nonspecific chronic low back pain? A systematic review of qualitative studies. *The Clinical Journal of Pain* **30**, 995–1005 (2014).

33. Pfingsten, M., *et al.* Fear-avoidance behavior and anticipation of pain in patients with chronic low back pain: A randomized controlled study. *Pain Medicine* **2**, 259–266 (2001).

34. Boudreau, M., *et al.* Impact of panic attacks on bronchoconstriction and subjective distress in asthma patients with and without panic disorder. *Psychosomatic Medicine* **79**, 576–584 (2017).

35. Witcraft, S.M., Dixon, L.J., Leukel, P. & Lee, A.A. Anxiety sensitivity and respiratory disease outcomes among individuals with chronic obstructive pulmonary disease. *General Hospital Psychiatry* **69**, 1–6 (2021).

36. van Tilburg, M.A., Palsson, O.S. & Whitehead, W.E. Which psychological factors exacerbate irritable bowel syndrome? Development of a comprehensive model. *Journal of Psychosomatic Research* **74**, 486–492 (2013).

37. Yoshino, A., *et al.* Sadness enhances the experience of pain via neural activation in the anterior cingulate cortex and amygdala: An fMRI study. *Neuroimage* **50**, 1194–1201 (2010).

38. Gray, K. & Wegner, D.M. The sting of intentional pain. *Psychological Science* **19**, 1260–1262 (2008).

39. Pfingsten, M., *et al.* Fear-avoidance behavior and anticipation of pain in patients with chronic low back pain: A randomized controlled study. *Pain Medicine* **2**, 259–266 (2001).

40. Pfingsten, M., *et al.* Fear-avoidance behavior and anticipation of pain in patients with chronic low back pain: A randomized controlled study. *Pain Medicine* **2**, 259–266 (2001).

41. Jamieson, J.P., Nock, M.K. & Mendes, W.B. Mind over matter: Reappraising arousal improves cardiovascular and cognitive responses to stress. *Journal of Experimental Psychology: General* **141**, 417 (2012).

42. Wood, J.V., Elaine Perunovic, W. & Lee, J.W. Positive self-statements: Power for some, peril for others. *Psychological Science* **20**, 860–866 (2009).

43. Symons, C.M., O'Sullivan, G.A. & Polman, R. The impacts of discriminatory experiences on lesbian, gay and bisexual people in sport. *Annals of Leisure Research* **20**, 467–489 (2017).

44. Caceres, B.A., *et al.* Assessing and addressing cardiovascular health in LGBTQ adults: A scientific statement from the American Heart Association. *Circulation* **142**, e321–e332 (2020).

45. Herrick, S.S. & Duncan, L.R. A systematic scoping review of engagement in physical activity among LGBTQ+ adults. *Journal of Physical Activity and Health* **15**, 226–232 (2018).

46. Meyer, M.L., Williams, K.D. & Eisenberger, N.I. Why social pain can live on: Different neural mechanisms are associated with reliving social and physical pain. *PLOS ONE* **10**, e0128294 (2015).

47. Eisenberger, N.I., Lieberman, M.D. & Williams, K.D. Does rejection hurt? An fMRI study of social exclusion. *Science* **302**, 290–292 (2003).

48. Meyer, M.L., Williams, K.D. & Eisenberger, N.I. Why social pain can live on: Different neural mechanisms are associated with reliving social and physical pain. *PLOS ONE* **10**, e0128294 (2015).

49. Danziger, N. & Willer, J.C. Tension-type headache as the unique pain experience of a patient with congenital insensitivity to pain. *Pain* **117**, 478–483 (2005).

50. Csupak, B., Sommer, J.L., Jacobsohn, E. & El-Gabalawy, R. A population-based examination of the co-occurrence and functional correlates of chronic pain and generalized anxiety disorder. *Journal of Anxiety Disorders* **56**, 74–80 (2018).

51. Doll, A., *et al.* Mindful attention to breath regulates emotions via increased amygdala–prefrontal cortex connectivity. *Neuroimage* **134**, 305–313 (2016).

52. Wells, R.E., *et al.* Attention to breath sensations does not engage endogenous opioids to reduce pain. *Pain* **161**, 1884–1893 (2020).

53. Shelov, D.V., Suchday, S. & Friedberg, J.P. A pilot study measuring the impact of yoga on the trait of mindfulness. *Behavioural and Cognitive Psychotherapy* **37**, 595 (2009).

54. Zhang, J., *et al.* A randomized controlled trial of mindfulness-based tai chi chuan for subthreshold depression adolescents. *Neuropsychiatric Disease and Treatment* **14**, 2313 (2018).

55. Caldwell, K., Adams, M., Quin, R., Harrison, M. & Greeson, J. Pilates, mindfulness and somatic education. *Journal of Dance & Somatic Practices* **5**, 141–153 (2013).

56. Mothes, H., Klaperski, S., Seelig, H., Schmidt, S. & Fuchs, R. Regular aerobic exercise increases dispositional mindfulness in men: A randomized controlled trial. *Mental Health and Physical Activity* **7**, 111–119 (2014).

57. Ulmer, C.S., Stetson, B.A. & Salmon, P.G. Mindfulness and acceptance are associated with exercise maintenance in YMCA exercisers. *Behaviour Research and Therapy* **48**, 805–809 (2010).

3. Mental Health Is Physical Health

1. Mojtabai, R. & Olfson, M. Proportion of antidepressants prescribed without a psychiatric diagnosis is growing. *Health Affairs* **30**, 1434–1442 (2011).

2. Spielmans, G.I., Spence-Sing, T. & Parry, P. Duty to warn: Antidepressant black box suicidality warning is empirically justified. *Frontiers in Psychiatry* **11**, 18 (2020).

3. Andrews, P.W. & Thomson Jr, J.A. The bright side of being blue: Depression as an adaptation for analyzing complex problems. *Psychological Review* **116**, 620 (2009).

4. Fava, M. & Davidson, K.G. Definition and epidemiology of treatment-resistant depression. *Psychiatric Clinics of North America* **19**, 179–200 (1996).

5. James, S.L., *et al.* Global, regional, and national incidence, prevalence, and years lived with disability for 354 diseases and injuries for 195 countries and territories, 1990–2017: A systematic analysis for the Global Burden of Disease Study 2017. *The Lancet* **392**, 1789–1858 (2018).

6. Santosh, P.J. & Malhotra, S. Varied psychiatric manifestations of acute intermittent porphyria. *Biological Psychiatry* **36**, 744–747 (1994).

7. Dienberg Love, G., Seeman, T.E., Weinstein, M. & Ryff, C.D. Bioindicators in the MIDUS national study: Protocol, measures, sample, and comparative context. *Journal of Aging and Health* **22**, 1059–1080 (2010).

8. Sin, N.L., Graham-Engeland, J.E., Ong, A.D. & Almeida, D.M. Affective reactivity to daily stressors is associated with elevated inflammation. *Health Psychology* **34**, 1154 (2015).

9. Charles, S.T., Piazza, J.R., Mogle, J., Sliwinski, M.J. & Almeida, D.M. The wear and tear of daily stressors on mental health. *Psychological Science* **24**, 733–741 (2013).

10. Chiang, J.J., Turiano, N.A., Mroczek, D.K. & Miller, G.E. Affective reactivity to daily stress and 20-year mortality risk in adults with chronic illness: Findings from the National Study of Daily Experiences. *Health Psychology* **37**, 170 (2018).

11. Caballero, B. The global epidemic of obesity: An overview. *Epidemiologic Reviews* **29**, 1–5 (2007).

12. Van Cauter, E., Spiegel, K., Tasali, E. & Leproult, R. Metabolic consequences of sleep and sleep loss. *Sleep Medicine* **9**, S23–S28 (2008).

13. Piercy, K.L., *et al.* The physical activity guidelines for Americans. *The Journal of the American Medical Association* **320**, 2020–2028 (2018).

14. Booth, F.W., Gordon, S.E., Carlson, C.J. & Hamilton, M.T. Waging war on modern chronic diseases: Primary prevention through exercise biology. *Journal of Applied Physiology* (2000).

15. World Health Organization. *Global Status Report on Noncommunicable Diseases 2014.* https://apps.who.int/iris/bitstream/handle/10665/148114/9789241564854_eng.pdf (2014).

16. Chen, G.Y. & Nuñez, G. Sterile inflammation: Sensing and reacting to damage. *Nature Reviews Immunology* **10**, 826–837 (2010).

17. Buret, A.G. How stress induces intestinal hypersensitivity. *The American Journal of Pathology* **168**, 3 (2006).

18. Yang, J., *et al.* Lactose intolerance in irritable bowel syndrome patients with diarrhoea: The roles of anxiety, activation of the innate mucosal immune system and visceral sensitivity. *Alimentary Pharmacology & Therapeutics* **39**, 302–311 (2014).

19. Chida, Y., Hamer, M. & Steptoe, A. A bidirectional relationship between psychosocial factors and atopic disorders: A systematic review and meta-analysis. *Psychosomatic Medicine* **70**, 102–116 (2008).

20. Pedersen, A., Zachariae, R. & Bovbjerg, D.H. Influence of psychological stress

on upper respiratory infection — a meta-analysis of prospective studies. *Psychosomatic Medicine* **72**, 823–832 (2010).

21. Kivimäki, M. & Kawachi, I. Work stress as a risk factor for cardiovascular disease. *Current Cardiology Reports* **17**, 1–9 (2015).

22. Sisó, S., Jeffrey, M. & González, L. Sensory circumventricular organs in health and disease. *Acta Neuropathologica* **120**, 689–705 (2010).

23. Savitz, J., *et al.* Putative neuroprotective and neurotoxic kynurenine pathway metabolites are associated with hippocampal and amygdalar volumes in subjects with major depressive disorder. *Neuropsychopharmacology* **40**, 463–471 (2015).

24. Couch, Y., *et al.* Microglial activation, increased TNF and SERT expression in the prefrontal cortex define stress-altered behaviour in mice susceptible to anhedonia. *Brain, Behavior, and Immunity* **29**, 136–146 (2013).

25. Lanquillon, S., Krieg, J.C., Bening-Abu-Shach, U. & Vedder, H. Cytokine production and treatment response in major depressive disorder. *Neuropsychopharmacology* **22**, 370–379 (2000).

26. Strawbridge, R., *et al.* Inflammation and clinical response to treatment in depression: A meta-analysis. *European Neuropsychopharmacology* **25**, 1532–1543 (2015).

27. Haroon, E., *et al.* Antidepressant treatment resistance is associated with increased inflammatory markers in patients with major depressive disorder. *Psychoneuroendocrinology* **95**, 43–49 (2018).

28. Svensson, T., *et al.* The association between complete and partial non-response to psychosocial questions and suicide: The JPHC Study. *The European Journal of Public Health* **25**, 424–430 (2015).

29. Rethorst, C.D., *et al.* Pro-inflammatory cytokines as predictors of antidepressant effects of exercise in major depressive disorder. *Molecular Psychiatry* **18**, 1119 (2013).

30. Corruble, E., Legrand, J., Duret, C., Charles, G. & Guelfi, J. IDS-C and IDS-sr: Psychometric properties in depressed in-patients. *Journal of Affective Disorders* **56**, 95–101 (1999).

31. Kvam, S., Kleppe, C.L., Nordhus, I.H. & Hovland, A. Exercise as a treatment for depression: A meta-analysis. *Journal of Affective Disorders* **202**, 67–86 (2016).

32. Schuch, F.B., *et al.* Exercise as a treatment for depression: A meta-analysis adjusting for publication bias. *Journal of Psychiatric Research* **77**, 42–51 (2016).

33. Netz, Y. Is the comparison between exercise and pharmacologic treatment of depression in the clinical practice guideline of the American College of Physicians evidence-based? *Frontiers in Pharmacology* **8**, 257 (2017).

34. Babyak, M., *et al.* Exercise treatment for major depression: Maintenance of therapeutic benefit at 10 months. *Psychosomatic Medicine* **62**, 633–638 (2000).

35. Das, A., *et al.* Comparison of treatment options for depression in heart

failure: A network meta-analysis. *Journal of Psychiatric Research* **108**, 7–23 (2019).

36. Thombs, B.D., *et al.* Does evidence support the American Heart Association's recommendation to screen patients for depression in cardiovascular care? An updated systematic review. *PLOS ONE* **8**, e52654 (2013).

37. Blumenthal, J.A., *et al.* Exercise and pharmacological treatment of depressive symptoms in patients with coronary heart disease: Results from the UPBEAT (Understanding the Prognostic Benefits of Exercise and Antidepressant Therapy) study. *Journal of the American College of Cardiology* **60**, 1053–1063 (2012).

38. Gleeson, M., *et al.* The anti-inflammatory effects of exercise: Mechanisms and implications for the prevention and treatment of disease. *Nature Reviews Immunology* **11**, 607–615 (2011).

39. Brandt, C. & Pedersen, B.K. The role of exercise-induced myokines in muscle homeostasis and the defense against chronic diseases. *Journal of Biomedicine and Biotechnology* **2010**, 1–6 (2010).

40. Severinsen, M.C.K. & Pedersen, B.K. Muscle–organ crosstalk: The emerging roles of myokines. *Endocrine Reviews* **41**, 594–609 (2020).

41. Champaneri, S., Wand, G.S., Malhotra, S.S., Casagrande, S.S. & Golden, S.H. Biological basis of depression in adults with diabetes. *Current Diabetes Reports* **10**, 396–405 (2010).

42. Nerurkar, L., Siebert, S., McInnes, I.B. & Cavanagh, J. Rheumatoid arthritis and depression: An inflammatory perspective. *The Lancet Psychiatry* **6**, 164–173 (2019).

43. Sforzini, L., Nettis, M.A., Mondelli, V. & Pariante, C.M. Inflammation in cancer and depression: A starring role for the kynurenine pathway. *Psychopharmacology*, 1–15 (2019).

44. Paolucci, E.M., Loukov, D., Bowdish, D.M. & Heisz, J.J. Exercise reduces depression and inflammation but intensity matters. *Biological Psychology* **133**, 79–84 (2018).

45. Gerritsen, R.J. & Band, G.P. Breath of life: The respiratory vagal stimulation model of contemplative activity. *Frontiers in Human Neuroscience* **12**, 397 (2018).

46. Buchheit, M., *et al.* Monitoring endurance running performance using cardiac parasympathetic function. *European Journal of Applied Physiology* **108**, 1153–1167 (2010).

47. Machhada, A., *et al.* Vagal determinants of exercise capacity. *Nature Communications* **8**, 1–7 (2017).

48. von Haaren, B., Haertel, S., Stumpp, J., Hey, S. & Ebner-Priemer, U. Reduced emotional stress reactivity to a real-life academic examination stressor in students participating in a 20-week aerobic exercise training: A randomised controlled trial using Ambulatory Assessment. *Psychology of Sport and Exercise* **20**, 67–75 (2015).

49. Netz, Y. Is the comparison between exercise and pharmacologic treatment of depression in the clinical practice guideline of the American College of Physicians evidence-based? *Frontiers in Pharmacology* **8**, 257 (2017).

50. Nebiker, L., *et al.* Moderating effects of exercise duration and intensity in neuromuscular vs. endurance exercise interventions for the treatment of depression: A meta-analytical review. *Frontiers in Psychiatry* **9**, 305 (2018).

51. Sabir, M.S., *et al.* Optimal vitamin D spurs serotonin: 1, 25-dihydroxyvitamin D represses serotonin reuptake transport (SERT) and degradation (MAO-A) gene expression in cultured rat serotonergic neuronal cell lines. *Genes & Nutrition* **13**, 19 (2018).

52. Parker, G.B., Brotchie, H. & Graham, R.K. Vitamin D and depression. *Journal of Affective Disorders* **208**, 56–61 (2017).

53. Harvey, S.B., *et al.* Exercise and the prevention of depression: Results of the HUNT cohort study. *American Journal of Psychiatry* **175**, 28–36 (2018).

54. Rector, N.A., Richter, M.A., Lerman, B. & Regev, R. A pilot test of the additive benefits of physical exercise to CBT for OCD. *Cognitive Behaviour Therapy* **44**, 328–340 (2015).

4. Free Yourself from Addiction

1. Mónok, K., *et al.* Psychometric properties and concurrent validity of two exercise addiction measures: A population wide study. *Psychology of Sport and Exercise* **13**, 739–746 (2012).

2. Sussman, S., Lisha, N. & Griffiths, M. Prevalence of the addictions: A problem of the majority or the minority? *Evaluation & the Health Professions* **34**, 3–56 (2011).

3. Trott, M., *et al.* Exercise addiction prevalence and correlates in the absence of eating disorder symptomology: A systematic review and meta-analysis. *Journal of Addiction Medicine* **14**, e321–e329 (2020).

4. Lichtenstein, M.B. & Jensen, T.T. Exercise addiction in CrossFit: Prevalence and psychometric properties of the Exercise Addiction Inventory. *Addictive Behaviors Reports* **3**, 33–37 (2016).

5. Herie, M., Godden, T., Shenfeld, J. & Kelly, C. *Addiction: An Information Guide.* Centre for Addiction and Mental Health. https://www.camh.ca/-/media/files/guides-and-publications/addiction-guide-en.pdf (2010).

6. Szabo, A., Griffiths, M.D., Marcos, R.d.L.V., Mervó, B. & Demetrovics, Z. Focus: Addiction: Methodological and conceptual limitations in exercise addiction research. *The Yale Journal of Biology and Medicine* **88**, 303 (2015).

7. Sutoo, D. & Akiyama, K. The mechanism by which exercise modifies brain function. *Physiology & Behavior* **60**, 177–181 (1996).

8. Hernandez, L. & Hoebel, B.G. Food reward and cocaine increase extracellular dopamine in the nucleus accumbens as measured by microdialysis. *Life Sciences* **42**, 1705–1712 (1988).

9. Fiorino, D.F. & Phillips, A.G. Facilitation of sexual behavior and enhanced

dopamine efflux in the nucleus accumbens of male rats after D-amphetamine-induced behavioral sensitization. *Journal of Neuroscience* **19**, 456–463 (1999).

10. Di Chiara, G. & Imperato, A. Drugs abused by humans preferentially increase synaptic dopamine concentrations in the mesolimbic system of freely moving rats. *Proceedings of the National Academy of Sciences* **85**, 5274–5278 (1988).

11. Volkow, N.D., Fowler, J.S., Wang, G.-J. & Swanson, J.M. Dopamine in drug abuse and addiction: Results from imaging studies and treatment implications. *Molecular Psychiatry* **9**, 557–569 (2004).

12. Krasnova, I.N., *et al.* Methamphetamine self-administration is associated with persistent biochemical alterations in striatal and cortical dopaminergic terminals in the rat. *PLOS ONE* **5**, e8790 (2010).

13. Ballard, M.E., *et al.* Low dopamine D2/D3 receptor availability is associated with steep discounting of delayed rewards in methamphetamine dependence. *International Journal of Neuropsychopharmacology* **18** (2015).

14. Cass, W.A. & Manning, M.W. Recovery of presynaptic dopaminergic functioning in rats treated with neurotoxic doses of methamphetamine. *Journal of Neuroscience* **19**, 7653–7660 (1999).

15. Woolverton, W.L., Ricaurte, G.A., Forno, L.S. & Seiden, L.S. Long-term effects of chronic methamphetamine administration in rhesus monkeys. *Brain Research* **486**, 73–78 (1989).

16. Wang, G., *et al.* Decreased dopamine activity predicts relapse in methamphetamine abusers. *Molecular Psychiatry* **17**, 918–925 (2012).

17. Sutoo, D. & Akiyama, K. The mechanism by which exercise modifies brain function. *Physiology & Behavior* **60**, 177–181 (1996).

18. Robertson, C.L., *et al.* Effect of exercise training on striatal dopamine D2/D3 receptors in methamphetamine users during behavioral treatment. *Neuropsychopharmacology* **41**, 1629–1636 (2016).

19. Goldfarb, A.H., Hatfield, B., Armstrong, D. & Potts, J. Plasma beta-endorphin concentration: Response to intensity and duration of exercise. *Medicine and Science in Sports and Exercise* **22**, 241–244 (1990).

20. Dietrich, A. & McDaniel, W.F. Endocannabinoids and exercise. *British Journal of Sports Medicine* **38**, 536–541 (2004).

21. Boecker, H., *et al.* The runner's high: Opioidergic mechanisms in the human brain. *Cerebral Cortex* **18**, 2523–2531 (2008).

22. Fuss, J., *et al.* A runner's high depends on cannabinoid receptors in mice. *Proceedings of the National Academy of Sciences* **112**, 13105–13108 (2015).

23. Raichlen, D.A., Foster, A.D., Seillier, A., Giuffrida, A. & Gerdeman, G.L. Exercise-induced endocannabinoid signaling is modulated by intensity. *European Journal of Applied Physiology* **113**, 869–875 (2013).

24. Dietrich, A. & McDaniel, W.F. Endocannabinoids and exercise. *British Journal of Sports Medicine* **38**, 536–541 (2004).

25. Mitchell, M.R., Berridge, K.C. & Mahler, S.V. Endocannabinoid-enhanced "liking" in nucleus accumbens shell hedonic hotspot requires endogenous opioid signals. *Cannabis and Cannabinoid Research* **3**, 166–170 (2018).

26. Schwarz, L. & Kindermann, W. β-Endorphin, catecholamines, and cortisol during exhaustive endurance exercise. *International Journal of Sports Medicine* **10**, 324–328 (1989).

27. Cohen, E.E., Ejsmond-Frey, R., Knight, N. & Dunbar, R.I. Rowers' high: Behavioural synchrony is correlated with elevated pain thresholds. *Biology Letters* **6**, 106–108 (2010).

28. Tarr, B., Launay, J., Cohen, E. & Dunbar, R. Synchrony and exertion during dance independently raise pain threshold and encourage social bonding. *Biology Letters* **11**, 2015.0767 (2015).

29. Sullivan, P. & Rickers, K. The effect of behavioral synchrony in groups of teammates and strangers. *International Journal of Sport and Exercise Psychology* **11**, 286–291 (2013).

30. Whiteman-Sandland, J., Hawkins, J. & Clayton, D. The role of social capital and community belongingness for exercise adherence: An exploratory study of the CrossFit gym model. *Journal of Health Psychology* **23**, 1545–1556 (2018).

31. Wise, R.A. Dopamine and reward: The anhedonia hypothesis 30 years on. *Neurotoxicity Research* **14**, 169–183 (2008).

32. Ferreri, L., *et al.* Dopamine modulates the reward experiences elicited by music. *Proceedings of the National Academy of Sciences* **116**, 3793–3798 (2019).

33. Wang, D., Wang, Y., Wang, Y., Li, R. & Zhou, C. Impact of physical exercise on substance use disorders: A meta-analysis. *PLOS ONE* **9**, e110728 (2014).

34. Mooney, L.J., *et al.* Exercise for methamphetamine dependence: Rationale, design, and methodology. *Contemporary Clinical Trials* **37**, 139–147 (2014).

35. Robertson, C.L., *et al.* Effect of exercise training on striatal dopamine D2/D3 receptors in methamphetamine users during behavioral treatment. *Neuropsychopharmacology* **41**, 1629–1636 (2016).

36. Rawson, R.A., *et al.* The impact of exercise on depression and anxiety symptoms among abstinent methamphetamine-dependent individuals in a residential treatment setting. *Journal of Substance Abuse Treatment* **57**, 36–40 (2015).

37. Rawson, R.A., *et al.* Impact of an exercise intervention on methamphetamine use outcomes post-residential treatment care. *Drug and Alcohol Dependence* **156**, 21–28 (2015).

38. Abrantes, A.M., *et al.* Exercise preferences of patients in substance abuse treatment. *Mental Health and Physical Activity* **4**, 79–87 (2011).

39. Beiter, R., Peterson, A., Abel, J. & Lynch, W. Exercise during early, but not late abstinence, attenuates subsequent relapse vulnerability in a rat model. *Translational Psychiatry* **6**, e792 (2016).

40. Robertson, C.L., *et al.* Effect of exercise training on striatal dopamine D2/D3 receptors in methamphetamine users during behavioral treatment. *Neuropsychopharmacology* **41**, 1629–1636 (2016).
41. Rawson, R.A., *et al.* Impact of an exercise intervention on methamphetamine use outcomes post-residential treatment care. *Drug and Alcohol Dependence* **156**, 21–28 (2015).
42. Goldstein, R.Z. & Volkow, N.D. Dysfunction of the prefrontal cortex in addiction: Neuroimaging findings and clinical implications. *Nature Reviews Neuroscience* **12**, 652–669 (2011).
43. Brecht, M.L. & Herbeck, D. Time to relapse following treatment for methamphetamine use: A long-term perspective on patterns and predictors. *Drug and Alcohol Dependence* **139**, 18–25 (2014).
44. Shin, C.B., *et al.* Incubation of cocaine-craving relates to glutamate over-flow within ventromedial prefrontal cortex. *Neuropharmacology* **102**, 103–110 (2016).
45. Parvaz, M.A., Moeller, S.J. & Goldstein, R.Z. Incubation of cue-induced craving in adults addicted to cocaine measured by electroencephalography. *The Journal of the American Medical Association Psychiatry* **73**, 1127–1134 (2016).
46. Abel, J.M., Nesil, T., Bakhti-Suroosh, A., Grant, P.A. & Lynch, W.J. Mechanisms underlying the efficacy of exercise as an intervention for cocaine relapse: A focus on mGlu5 in the dorsal medial prefrontal cortex. *Psychopharmacology*, 1–17 (2019).
47. Wang, D., Zhou, C., Zhao, M., Wu, X. & Chang, Y.-K. Dose–response relationships between exercise intensity, cravings, and inhibitory control in methamphetamine dependence: An ERPs study. *Drug and Alcohol Dependence* **161**, 331–339 (2016).
48. Wang, D., Zhu, T., Zhou, C. & Chang, Y.-K. Aerobic exercise training ameliorates craving and inhibitory control in methamphetamine dependencies: A randomized controlled trial and event-related potential study. *Psychology of Sport and Exercise* **30**, 82–90 (2017).
49. Lautner, S.C., Patterson, M.S., Ramirez, M. & Heinrich, K. Can CrossFit aid in addiction recovery? An exploratory media analysis of popular press. *Mental Health and Social Inclusion* **24** (2020).
50. Bava, S. & Tapert, S.F. Adolescent brain development and the risk for alcohol and other drug problems. *Neuropsychology Review* **20**, 398–413 (2010).
51. Galvan, A. Adolescent development of the reward system. *Frontiers in Human Neuroscience* **4**, 6 (2010).
52. Hill, S.Y., *et al.* Dopaminergic mutations: Within-family association and linkage in multiplex alcohol dependence families. *American Journal of Medical Genetics Part B: Neuropsychiatric Genetics* **147**, 517–526 (2008).
53. Giacometti, L. & Barker, J. Sex differences in the glutamate system: Implications for addiction. *Neuroscience & Biobehavioral Reviews* **113**, 157–168 (2020).

54. Bobzean, S.A., DeNobrega, A.K. & Perrotti, L.I. Sex differences in the neuro-biology of drug addiction. *Experimental Neurology* **259**, 64–74 (2014).

55. Velicer, W.F., *et al.* Multiple behavior interventions to prevent substance abuse and increase energy balance behaviors in middle school students. *Translational Behavioral Medicine* **3**, 82–93 (2013).

56. Korhonen, T., Kujala, U.M., Rose, R.J. & Kaprio, J. Physical activity in ado-lescence as a predictor of alcohol and illicit drug use in early adulthood: A longitudinal population-based twin study. *Twin Research and Human Genetics* **12**, 261–268 (2009).

57. Cooper, A.R., *et al.* Objectively measured physical activity and sedentary time in youth: The International Children's Accelerometry Database (ICAD). *International Journal of Behavioral Nutrition and Physical Activity* **12**, 1–10 (2015).

58. García-Rodríguez, O., *et al.* Probability and predictors of relapse to smoking: Results of the National Epidemiologic Survey on Alcohol and Related Condi-tions (NESARC). *Drug and Alcohol Dependence* **132**, 479–485 (2013).

59. Campana, B., Brasiel, P.G., de Aguiar, A.S. & Dutra, S.C.P.L. Obesity and food addiction: Similarities to drug addiction. *Obesity Medicine* **16**, 100136 (2019).

60. Mantsch, J.R., Baker, D.A., Funk, D., Lê, A.D. & Shaham, Y. Stress-induced reinstatement of drug seeking: 20 years of progress. *Neuropsychopharmacol-ogy* **41**, 335 (2016).

5. Keep Your Brain Young

1. Mendonça, J., Marques, S. & Abrams, D. Children's attitudes toward older people: Current and future directions. *Contemporary Perspectives on Ageism*, 517–548 (2018).

2. Mendonça, J., Marques, S. & Abrams, D. Children's attitudes toward older people: Current and future directions. *Contemporary Perspectives on Ageism*, 517–548 (2018).

3. Levy, B.R. Mind matters: Cognitive and physical effects of aging self-stereotypes. *The Journals of Gerontology Series B: Psychological Sciences and Social Sciences* **58**, P203–P211 (2003).

4. Hess, T.M., Hinson, J.T. & Hodges, E.A. Moderators of and mechanisms un-derlying stereotype threat effects on older adults' memory performance. *Ex-perimental Aging Research* **35**, 153–177 (2009).

5. Hausdorff, J.M., Levy, B.R. & Wei, J.Y. The power of ageism on physical func-tion of older persons: Reversibility of age-related gait changes. *Journal of the American Geriatrics Society* **47**, 1346–1349 (1999).

6. Fenesi, B., *et al.* Physical exercise moderates the relationship of apolipopro-tein E (APOE) genotype and dementia risk: A population-based study. *Jour-nal of Alzheimer's Disease* **56**, 297–303 (2017).

7. Edwardson, C.L., *et al.* Association of sedentary behaviour with metabolic syndrome: A meta-analysis. *PLOS ONE* **7**, e34916 (2012).

8. Verhaaren, B.F., *et al.* High blood pressure and cerebral white matter lesion progression in the general population. *Hypertension* **61**, 1354–1359 (2013).

9. Vermeer, S.E., *et al.* Silent brain infarcts and white matter lesions increase stroke risk in the general population: The Rotterdam Scan Study. *Stroke* **34**, 1126–1129 (2003).

10. Debette, S. & Markus, H. The clinical importance of white matter hyperintensities on brain magnetic resonance imaging: Systematic review and meta-analysis. *The British Medical Journal* **341** (2010).

11. Gorelick, P.B., *et al.* Vascular contributions to cognitive impairment and dementia: A statement for healthcare professionals from the American Heart Association/American Stroke Association. *Stroke* **42**, 2672–2713 (2011).

12. Emrani, S., *et al.* Alzheimer's/vascular spectrum dementia: Classification in addition to diagnosis. *Journal of Alzheimer's Disease* **73**, 63–71 (2020).

13. Perosa, V., *et al.* Hippocampal vascular reserve associated with cognitive performance and hippocampal volume. *Brain* **143**, 622–634 (2020).

14. de La Torre, J.C. Alzheimer's disease is a vasocognopathy: A new term to describe its nature. *Neurological Research* **26**, 517–524 (2004).

15. Yan, S., *et al.* Association between sedentary behavior and the risk of dementia: A systematic review and meta-analysis. *Translational Psychiatry* **10**, 1–8 (2020).

16. van Alphen, H.J., *et al.* Older adults with dementia are sedentary for most of the day. *PLOS ONE* **11**, e0152457 (2016).

17. Carter, S.E., *et al.* Regular walking breaks prevent the decline in cerebral blood flow associated with prolonged sitting. *Journal of Applied Physiology* **125**, 790–798 (2018).

18. Loh, R., Stamatakis, E., Folkerts, D., Allgrove, J.E. & Moir, H.J. Effects of interrupting prolonged sitting with physical activity breaks on blood glucose, insulin and triacylglycerol measures: A systematic review and meta-analysis. *Sports Medicine* **50**, 295–330 (2020).

19. Ekelund, U., *et al.* Does physical activity attenuate, or even eliminate, the detrimental association of sitting time with mortality? A harmonised meta-analysis of data from more than 1 million men and women. *The Lancet* **388**, 1302–1310 (2016).

20. Mckendry, J., Breen, L., Shad, B.J. & Greig, C.A. Muscle morphology and performance in master athletes: A systematic review and meta-analyses. *Ageing Research Reviews* **45**, 62–82 (2018).

21. Kontro, T.K., Sarna, S., Kaprio, J. & Kujala, U.M. Mortality and health-related habits in 900 Finnish former elite athletes and their brothers. *British Journal of Sports Medicine* **52**, 89–95 (2018).

22. Rogers, M.A., Hagberg, J.M., Martin 3rd, W., Ehsani, A. & Holloszy, J.O. De-

cline in VO2 max with aging in master athletes and sedentary men. *Journal of Applied Physiology* **68**, 2195–2199 (1990).

23. Kurl, S., Laukkanen, J., Lonnroos, E., Remes, A. & Soininen, H. Cardiorespiratory fitness and risk of dementia: A prospective population-based cohort study. *Age and Ageing* **47**, 611–614 (2018).

24. Hörder, H., *et al.* Midlife cardiovascular fitness and dementia: A 44-year longitudinal population study in women. *Neurology* **90**, e1298–e1305 (2018).

25. Lalande, S., *et al.* Effects of interval walking on physical fitness in middle-aged individuals. *Journal of Primary Care & Community Health* **1**, 104–110 (2010).

26. Morikawa, M., *et al.* Physical fitness and indices of lifestyle-related diseases before and after interval walking training in middle-aged and older males and females. *British Journal of Sports Medicine* **45**, 216–224 (2011).

27. Karstoft, K., *et al.* The effects of free-living interval-walking training on glycemic control, body composition, and physical fitness in type 2 diabetic patients: A randomized, controlled trial. *Diabetes Care* **36**, 228–236 (2013).

28. Lachman, M.E. Development in midlife. *The Annual Review of Psychology* **55**, 305–331 (2004).

29. Reed, J.L. & Pipe, A.L. The talk test: A useful tool for prescribing and monitoring exercise intensity. *Current Opinion in Cardiology* **29**, 475–480 (2014).

30. Stienen, M.N., *et al.* Reliability of the 6-minute walking test smartphone application. *Journal of Neurosurgery: Spine* **31**, 786–793 (2019).

31. Burr, J.F., Bredin, S.S., Faktor, M.D. & Warburton, D.E. The 6-minute walk test as a predictor of objectively measured aerobic fitness in healthy working-aged adults. *The Physician and Sports Medicine* **39**, 133–139 (2011).

32. Kurl, S., Laukkanen, J., Lonnroos, E., Remes, A. & Soininen, H. Cardiorespiratory fitness and risk of dementia: A prospective population-based cohort study. *Age and Ageing* **47**, 611–614 (2018).

33. Ainslie, P.N., *et al.* Elevation in cerebral blood flow velocity with aerobic fitness throughout healthy human ageing. *The Journal of Physiology* **586**, 4005–4010 (2008).

34. Morland, C., *et al.* Exercise induces cerebral VEGF and angiogenesis via the lactate receptor HCAR1. *Nature Communications* **8**, 15557 (2017).

35. El Hayek, L., *et al.* Lactate mediates the effects of exercise on learning and memory through SIRT1-dependent activation of hippocampal brain-derived neurotrophic factor (BDNF). *Journal of Neuroscience* **39**, 2369–2382 (2019).

36. Phillips, H.S., *et al.* BDNF mRNA is decreased in the hippocampus of individuals with Alzheimer's disease. *Neuron* **7**, 695–702 (1991).

37. Altman, J. & Das, G.D. Autoradiographic and histological evidence of postnatal hippocampal neurogenesis in rats. *Journal of Comparative Neurology* **124**, 319–335 (1965).

38. Van Praag, H., Kempermann, G. & Gage, F.H. Running increases cell proliferation and neurogenesis in the adult mouse dentate gyrus. *Nature Neuroscience* **2**, 266 (1999).

39. Van Praag, H., Christie, B.R., Sejnowski, T.J. & Gage, F.H. Running enhances neurogenesis, learning, and long-term potentiation in mice. *Proceedings of the National Academy of Sciences* **96**, 13427–13431 (1999).

40. Van Praag, H., Kempermann, G. & Gage, F.H. Running increases cell proliferation and neurogenesis in the adult mouse dentate gyrus. *Nature Neuroscience* **2**, 266 (1999).

41. Van Praag, H., Christie, B.R., Sejnowski, T.J. & Gage, F.H. Running enhances neurogenesis, learning, and long-term potentiation in mice. *Proceedings of the National Academy of Sciences* **96**, 13427–13431 (1999).

42. Van Praag, H., Shubert, T., Zhao, C. & Gage, F.H. Exercise enhances learning and hippocampal neurogenesis in aged mice. *Journal of Neuroscience* **25**, 8680–8685 (2005).

43. Boldrini, M., *et al.* Human hippocampal neurogenesis persists throughout aging. *Cell Stem Cell* **22**, 589–599. e585 (2018).

44. Sorrells, S.F., *et al.* Human hippocampal neurogenesis drops sharply in children to undetectable levels in adults. *Nature* **555**, 377 (2018).

45. Jack, C., *et al.* Rate of medial temporal lobe atrophy in typical aging and Alzheimer's disease. *Neurology* **51**, 993–999 (1998).

46. Erickson, K.I., *et al.* Exercise training increases size of hippocampus and improves memory. *Proceedings of the National Academy of Sciences* **108**, 3017–3022 (2011).

47. Maass, A., *et al.* Vascular hippocampal plasticity after aerobic exercise in older adults. *Molecular Psychiatry* **20**, 585–593 (2015).

48. Gorbach, T., *et al.* Longitudinal association between hippocampus atrophy and episodic-memory decline. *Neurobiology of Aging* **51**, 167–176 (2017).

49. Tromp, D., Dufour, A., Lithfous, S., Pebayle, T. & Després, O. Episodic memory in normal aging and Alzheimer disease: Insights from imaging and behavioral studies. *Ageing Research Reviews* **24**, 232–262 (2015).

50. Kovacevic, A., Fenesi, B., Paolucci, E. & Heisz, J.J. The effects of aerobic exercise intensity on memory in older adults. *Applied Physiology, Nutrition, and Metabolism* (2019).

51. Lourenco, M.V., *et al.* Cerebrospinal fluid irisin correlates with amyloid-β, BDNF, and cognition in Alzheimer's disease. *Alzheimer's & Dementia: Diagnosis, Assessment & Disease Monitoring* **12**, e12034 (2020).

52. Lourenco, M.V., *et al.* Exercise-linked FNDC5/irisin rescues synaptic plasticity and memory defects in Alzheimer's models. *Nature Medicine* **25**, 165 (2019).

53. Lourenco, M.V., *et al.* Cerebrospinal fluid irisin correlates with amyloid-β, BDNF, and cognition in Alzheimer's disease. *Alzheimer's & Dementia: Diagnosis, Assessment & Disease Monitoring* **12**, e12034 (2020).

54. de Freitas, G.B., Lourenco, M.V. & De Felice, F.G. Protective actions of exercise-related FNDC5/Irisin in memory and Alzheimer's disease. *Journal of Neurochemistry* **155**, 602–611 (2020).

55. Okwumabua, T.M., Meyers, A.W. & Santille, L. A demographic and cognitive profile of master runners. *Journal of Sport Behavior* **10**, 212 (1987).

56. Frisoni, G.B., *et al.* Mild cognitive impairment in the population and physical health: Data on 1,435 individuals aged 75 to 95. *The Journals of Gerontology Series A: Biological Sciences and Medical Sciences* **55**, M322–M328 (2000).

57. Sachdev, P.S., *et al.* Factors predicting reversion from mild cognitive impairment to normal cognitive functioning: A population-based study. *PLOS ONE* **8**, e59649 (2013).

58. Singh, M.A.F., *et al.* The Study of Mental and Resistance Training (SMART) study — resistance training and/or cognitive training in mild cognitive impairment: A randomized, double-blind, double-sham controlled trial. *Journal of the American Medical Directors Association* **15**, 873–880 (2014).

59. Tak, E.C., van Uffelen, J.G., Paw, M.J.C.A., van Mechelen, W. & Hopman-Rock, M. Adherence to exercise programs and determinants of maintenance in older adults with mild cognitive impairment. *Journal of Aging and Physical Activity* **20**, 32–46 (2012).

60. Penninkilampi, R., Casey, A.-N., Singh, M.F. & Brodaty, H. The association between social engagement, loneliness, and risk of dementia: A systematic review and meta-analysis. *Journal of Alzheimer's Disease* **66**, 1619–1633 (2018).

61. Sundström, A., Adolfsson, A.N., Nordin, M. & Adolfsson, R. Loneliness increases the risk of all-cause dementia and Alzheimer's disease. *The Journals of Gerontology: Series B* **75**, 919–926 (2020).

62. Dunlop, W.L. & Beauchamp, M.R. Birds of a feather stay active together: A case study of an all-male older adult exercise program. *Journal of Aging and Physical Activity* **21**, 222–232 (2013).

63. Farrance, C., Tsofliou, F. & Clark, C. Adherence to community based group exercise interventions for older people: A mixed-methods systematic review. *Preventive Medicine* **87**, 155–166 (2016).

64. Kanamori, S., *et al.* Exercising alone versus with others and associations with subjective health status in older Japanese: The JAGES Cohort Study. *Scientific Reports* **6**, 1–7 (2016).

65. Brady, S., *et al.* Reducing isolation and loneliness through membership in a fitness program for older adults: Implications for health. *Journal of Applied Gerontology* **39**, 301–310 (2020).

66. Hawkley, L.C. & Cacioppo, J.T. Loneliness matters: A theoretical and empirical review of consequences and mechanisms. *Annals of Behavioral Medicine* **40**, 218–227 (2010).

67. Hawkley, L.C., Thisted, R.A. & Cacioppo, J.T. Loneliness predicts reduced physical activity: Cross-sectional & longitudinal analyses. *Health Psychology* **28**, 354 (2009).

68. Devereux-Fitzgerald, A., Powell, R., Dewhurst, A. & French, D.P. The accept-

ability of physical activity interventions to older adults: A systematic review and meta-synthesis. *Social Science & Medicine* **158**, 14–23 (2016).

69. Stubbs, B., *et al.* Risk of hospitalized falls and hip fractures in 22,103 older adults receiving mental health care vs 161,603 controls: A large cohort study. *Journal of the American Medical Directors Association* **21**, 1893–1899 (2020).

70. Karssemeijer, E.G., *et al.* Exergaming as a physical exercise strategy reduces frailty in people with dementia: A randomized controlled trial. *Journal of the American Medical Directors Association* **20**, 1502–1508. e1501 (2019).

71. Northey, J.M., Cherbuin, N., Pumpa, K.L., Smee, D.J. & Rattray, B. Exercise interventions for cognitive function in adults older than 50: A systematic review with meta-analysis. *British Journal of Sports Medicine* **52**, 154–160 (2018).

6. Move More to Sleep, Think, and Feel Better

1. Roth, T. Insomnia: Definition, prevalence, etiology, and consequences. *Journal of Clinical Sleep Medicine* **3**, S7–S10 (2007).

2. Timpano, K.R., Carbonella, J.Y., Bernert, R.A. & Schmidt, N.B. Obsessive compulsive symptoms and sleep difficulties: Exploring the unique relationship between insomnia and obsessions. *Journal of Psychiatric Research* **57**, 101–107 (2014).

3. Morin, C.M., *et al.* Insomnia disorder. *Nature Reviews Disease Primers* **1**, 1–18 (2015).

4. Hirshkowitz, M., *et al.* National Sleep Foundation's sleep time duration recommendations: Methodology and results summary. *Sleep Health* **1**, 40–43 (2015).

5. Olds, T., Blunden, S., Petkov, J. & Forchino, F. The relationships between sex, age, geography and time in bed in adolescents: A meta-analysis of data from 23 countries. *Sleep Medicine Reviews* **14**, 371–378 (2010).

6. Dregan, A. & Armstrong, D. Adolescence sleep disturbances as predictors of adulthood sleep disturbances — a cohort study. *Journal of Adolescent Health* **46**, 482–487 (2010).

7. Cohen, D.A., *et al.* Uncovering residual effects of chronic sleep loss on human performance. *Science Translational Medicine* **2**, 14ra13 (2010).

8. Taylor, D.J., Lichstein, K.L., Durrence, H.H., Reidel, B.W. & Bush, A.J. Epidemiology of insomnia, depression, and anxiety. *Sleep* **28**, 1457–1464 (2005).

9. Shao, Y., *et al.* Altered resting-state amygdala functional connectivity after 36 hours of total sleep deprivation. *PLOS ONE* **9**, e112222 (2014).

10. Jamieson, D., Broadhouse, K.M., Lagopoulos, J. & Hermens, D.F. Investigating the links between adolescent sleep deprivation, fronto-limbic connectivity and the onset of mental disorders: A review of the literature. *Sleep Medicine* **66**, 61–67 (2020).

11. Baum, K.T., *et al.* Sleep restriction worsens mood and emotion regulation in adolescents. *Journal of Child Psychology and Psychiatry* **55**, 180–190 (2014).

12. Wong, M.M., Brower, K.J. & Zucker, R.A. Sleep problems, suicidal ideation, and self-harm behaviors in adolescence. *Journal of Psychiatric Research* **45**, 505–511 (2011).

13. https://www.nimh.nih.gov/health/statistics/suicide.

14. Krause, A.J., *et al.* The sleep-deprived human brain. *Nature Reviews Neuroscience* **18**, 404 (2017).

15. Poudel, G.R., Innes, C.R., Bones, P.J., Watts, R. & Jones, R.D. Losing the struggle to stay awake: Divergent thalamic and cortical activity during microsleeps. *Human Brain Mapping* **35**, 257–269 (2014).

16. Lo, J.C., Ong, J.L., Leong, R.L., Gooley, J.J. & Chee, M.W. Cognitive performance, sleepiness, and mood in partially sleep deprived adolescents: The Need for Sleep Study. *Sleep* **39**, 687–698 (2016).

17. Tefft, B.C. Asleep at the wheel: The prevalence and impact of drowsy driving. https://aaafoundation.org/wp-content/uploads/2018/02/2010DrowsyDrivingReport.pdf (2010).

18. Williamson, A.M. & Feyer, A.-M. Moderate sleep deprivation produces impairments in cognitive and motor performance equivalent to legally prescribed levels of alcohol intoxication. *Occupational and Environmental Medicine* **57**, 649–655 (2000).

19. Landrigan, C.P., *et al.* Effect of reducing interns' work hours on serious medical errors in intensive care units. *New England Journal of Medicine* **351**, 1838–1848 (2004).

20. Bromley, L.E., Booth III, J.N., Kilkus, J.M., Imperial, J.G. & Penev, P.D. Sleep restriction decreases the physical activity of adults at risk for type 2 diabetes. *Sleep* **35**, 977–984 (2012).

21. Taheri, S. The link between short sleep duration and obesity: We should recommend more sleep to prevent obesity. *Archives of Disease in Childhood* **91**, 881–884 (2006).

22. Knutson, K.L., Spiegel, K., Penev, P. & Van Cauter, E. The metabolic consequences of sleep deprivation. *Sleep Medicine Reviews* **11**, 163–178 (2007).

23. Kovacevic, A., Mavros, Y., Heisz, J.J. & Singh, M.A.F. The effect of resistance exercise on sleep: A systematic review of randomized controlled trials. *Sleep Medicine Reviews* **39**, 52–68 (2018).

24. Wang, W.L., Chen, K.H., Pan, Y.C., Yang, S.N. & Chan, Y.Y. The effect of yoga on sleep quality and insomnia in women with sleep problems: A systematic review and meta-analysis. *The British Medical Journal Psychiatry* **20**, 1–19 (2020).

25. Raman, G., Zhang, Y., Minichiello, V.J., D'Ambrosio, C.M. & Wang, C. Tai chi improves sleep quality in healthy adults and patients with chronic conditions: A systematic review and meta-analysis. *Journal of Sleep Disorders & Therapy* **2** (2013).

26. Kredlow, M.A., Capozzoli, M.C., Hearon, B.A., Calkins, A.W. & Otto, M.W.

The effects of physical activity on sleep: A meta-analytic review. *Journal of Behavioral Medicine* **38**, 427–449 (2015).

27. Czeisler, C.A., *et al.* Stability, precision, and near-24-hour period of the human circadian pacemaker. *Science* **284**, 2177–2181 (1999).

28. Daan, S. & Gwinner, E. Jürgen Aschoff (1913–98). *Nature* **396**, 418–418 (1998).

29. Aschoff, J. Circadian rhythms in man. *Science* **148**, 1427–1432 (1965).

30. Grivas, T.B. & Savvidou, O.D. Melatonin the "light of night" in human biology and adolescent idiopathic scoliosis. *Scoliosis* **2**, 6 (2007).

31. Haim, A. & Zubidat, A.E. Artificial light at night: Melatonin as a mediator between the environment and epigenome. *Philosophical Transactions of the Royal Society B: Biological Sciences* **370**, 20140121 (2015).

32. Lanfumey, L., Mongeau, R. & Hamon, M. Biological rhythms and melatonin in mood disorders and their treatments. *Pharmacology & Therapeutics* **138**, 176–184 (2013).

33. Youngstedt, S.D., *et al.* Circadian phase-shifting effects of bright light, exercise, and bright light + exercise. *Journal of Circadian Rhythms* **14** (2016).

34. Fischer, D., Lombardi, D.A., Marucci-Wellman, H. & Roenneberg, T. Chronotypes in the US — influence of age and sex. *PLOS ONE* **12**, e0178782 (2017).

35. Youngstedt, S.D., Elliott, J.A. & Kripke, D.F. Human circadian phase–response curves for exercise. *The Journal of Physiology* **597**, 2253–2268 (2019).

36. Kalak, N., *et al.* Daily morning running for 3 weeks improved sleep and psychological functioning in healthy adolescents compared with controls. *Journal of Adolescent Health* **51**, 615–622 (2012).

37. Stutz, J., Eiholzer, R. & Spengler, C.M. Effects of evening exercise on sleep in healthy participants: A systematic review and meta-analysis. *Sports Medicine* **49**, 269–287 (2019).

38. Oda, S. & Shirakawa, K. Sleep onset is disrupted following pre-sleep exercise that causes large physiological excitement at bedtime. *European Journal of Applied Physiology* **114**, 1789–1799 (2014).

39. Vogel, C., Wolpert, C. & Wehling, M. How to measure heart rate? *European Journal of Clinical Pharmacology* **60**, 461–466 (2004).

40. Nanchen, D. Resting heart rate: What is normal? *Heart* **104**, 1048–1049 (2018).

41. Lader, M. & Mathews, A. Physiological changes during spontaneous panic attacks. *Journal of Psychosomatic Research* **14**, 377–382 (1970).

42. Horváth, A., *et al.* Effects of state and trait anxiety on sleep structure: A polysomnographic study in 1083 subjects. *Psychiatry Research* **244**, 279–283 (2016).

43. Erlacher, D., Ehrlenspiel, F., Adegbesan, O.A. & Galal El-Din, H. Sleep habits in German athletes before important competitions or games. *Journal of Sports Sciences* **29**, 859–866 (2011).

44. Lowe, H., *et al.* Does exercise improve sleep for adults with insomnia? A

systematic review with quality appraisal. *Clinical Psychology Review* **68**, 1–12 (2019).

45. Baron, K.G., Reid, K.J. & Zee, P.C. Exercise to improve sleep in insomnia: Exploration of the bidirectional effects. *Journal of Clinical Sleep Medicine* **9**, 819–824 (2013).

46. Bastien, C.H., Vallières, A. & Morin, C.M. Validation of the Insomnia Severity Index as an outcome measure for insomnia research. *Sleep Medicine* **2**, 297–307 (2001).

47. Hartescu I., Morgan K. & Stevinson C.D. Increased physical activity improves sleep and mood outcomes in inactive people with insomnia: A randomized controlled trial. *Journal of Sleep Research* **24**, 526–534 (2015).

48. Kredlow, M.A., Capozzoli, M.C., Hearon, B.A., Calkins, A.W. & Otto, M.W. The effects of physical activity on sleep: A meta-analytic review. *Journal of Behavioral Medicine* **38**, 427–449 (2015).

49. Porkka-Heiskanen, T. & Kalinchuk, A.V. Adenosine, energy metabolism and sleep homeostasis. *Sleep Medicine Reviews* **15**, 123–135 (2011).

50. Dworak, M., Diel, P., Voss, S., Hollmann, W. & Strüder, H. Intense exercise increases adenosine concentrations in rat brain: Implications for a homeostatic sleep drive. *Neuroscience* **150**, 789–795 (2007).

51. Peng, W., *et al.* Regulation of sleep homeostasis mediator adenosine by basal forebrain glutamatergic neurons. *Science* **369** (2020).

52. Aschoff, J. Circadian rhythms in man. *Science* **148**, 1427–1432 (1965).

53. NASA. *Apollo 11 Mission Report*. https://www.nasa.gov/specials/apollo50th/pdf/A11_MissionReport.pdf

54. Cheng, W.J. & Cheng, Y. Night shift and rotating shift in association with sleep problems, burnout and minor mental disorder in male and female employees. *Occupational and Environmental Medicine* **74**, 483–488 (2017).

55. Porkka-Heiskanen, T. & Kalinchuk, A.V. Adenosine, energy metabolism and sleep homeostasis. *Sleep Medicine Reviews* **15**, 123–135 (2011).

56. Roehrs, T. & Roth, T. Caffeine: Sleep and daytime sleepiness. *Sleep Medicine Reviews* **12**, 153–162 (2008).

57. Van Dongen, H.P., Rogers, N.L. & Dinges, D.F. Sleep debt: Theoretical and empirical issues. *Sleep and Biological Rhythms* **1**, 5–13 (2003).

58. Spiegel, K., Leproult, R. & Van Cauter, E. Impact of sleep debt on metabolic and endocrine function. *The Lancet* **354**, 1435–1439 (1999).

59. Montagna, P. Fatal familial insomnia: A model disease in sleep physiopathology. *Sleep Medicine Reviews* **9**, 339–353 (2005).

60. Carskadon, M.A. & Dement, W.C. Normal human sleep: An overview. *Principles and Practice of Sleep Medicine* **4**, 13–23 (2005).

61. Montagna, P. Fatal familial insomnia: A model disease in sleep physiopathology. *Sleep Medicine Reviews* **9**, 339–353 (2005).

62. Fultz, N.E., *et al.* Coupled electrophysiological, hemodynamic, and cerebrospinal fluid oscillations in human sleep. *Science* **366**, 628–631 (2019).

63. Shapiro, C.M., Bortz, R., Mitchell, D., Bartel, P. & Jooste, P. Slow-wave sleep: A recovery period after exercise. *Science* **214**, 1253–1254 (1981).

64. Shapiro, C.M., Griesel, R.D., Bartel, P.R. & Jooste, P.L. Sleep patterns after graded exercise. *Journal of Applied Physiology* **39**, 187–190 (1975).

65. Martin, J.M., *et al.* Structural differences between REM and non-REM dream reports assessed by graph analysis. *PLOS ONE* **15**, e0228903 (2020).

66. Ohayon, M.M., Carskadon, M.A., Guilleminault, C. & Vitiello, M.V. Meta-analysis of quantitative sleep parameters from childhood to old age in healthy individuals: Developing normative sleep values across the human lifespan. *Sleep* **27**, 1255–1273 (2004).

67. Lee, Y.F., Gerashchenko, D., Timofeev, I., Bacskai, B.J. & Kastanenka, K.V. Slow wave sleep is a promising intervention target for Alzheimer's disease. *Frontiers in Neuroscience* **14** (2020).

68. Ju, Y.E.S., Lucey, B.P. & Holtzman, D.M. Sleep and Alzheimer disease pathology — a bidirectional relationship. *Nature Reviews Neurology* **10**, 115–119 (2014).

69. Yang, P.Y., Ho, K.H., Chen, H.C. & Chien, M.Y. Exercise training improves sleep quality in middle-aged and older adults with sleep problems: A systematic review. *Journal of Physiotherapy* **58**, 157–163 (2012).

70. Rupp, T.L., Wesensten, N.J., Bliese, P.D. & Balkin, T.J. Banking sleep: Realization of benefits during subsequent sleep restriction and recovery. *Sleep* **32**, 311–321 (2009).

71. Ebrahim, I.O., Shapiro, C.M., Williams, A.J. & Fenwick, P.B. Alcohol and sleep I: Effects on normal sleep. *Alcoholism: Clinical and Experimental Research* **37**, 539–549 (2013).

72. Wassing, R., *et al.* Restless REM sleep impedes overnight amygdala adaptation. *Current Biology* **29**, 2351–2358. e2354 (2019).

73. Wassing, R., *et al.* Haunted by the past: Old emotions remain salient in insomnia disorder. *Brain* **142**, 1783–1796 (2019).

74. Habukawa, M., *et al.* Differences in rapid eye movement (REM) sleep abnormalities between posttraumatic stress disorder (PTSD) and major depressive disorder patients: REM interruption correlated with nightmare complaints in PTSD. *Sleep Medicine* **43**, 34–39 (2018).

75. Schuckit, M.A. & Hesselbrock, V. Alcohol dependence and anxiety disorders: What is the relationship? *The American Journal of Psychiatry* **151**, 1723-1734 (1994).

76. Ebrahim, I.O., Shapiro, C.M., Williams, A.J. & Fenwick, P.B. Alcohol and sleep I: Effects on normal sleep. *Alcoholism: Clinical and Experimental Research* **37**, 539–549 (2013).

77. Pietilä, J., *et al.* Acute effect of alcohol intake on cardiovascular autonomic regulation during the first hours of sleep in a large real-world sample of Finnish employees: Observational study. *The Journal of Medical Internet Research Mental Health* **5**, e9519 (2018).

7. Staying Focused, Being Creative, and Sticking to It

1. Pattabiraman, K., Muchnik, S.K. & Sestan, N. The evolution of the human brain and disease susceptibility. *Current Opinion in Genetics & Development* **65**, 91–97 (2020).

2. Zbozinek, T.D., *et al.* Diagnostic overlap of generalized anxiety disorder and major depressive disorder in a primary care sample. *Depression and Anxiety* **29**, 1065–1071 (2012).

3. Bechara, A. Decision making, impulse control and loss of willpower to resist drugs: A neurocognitive perspective. *Nature Neuroscience* **8**, 1458–1463 (2005).

4. Chadick, J.Z., Zanto, T.P. & Gazzaley, A. Structural and functional differences in medial prefrontal cortex underlie distractibility and suppression deficits in ageing. *Nature Communications* **5**, 1–12 (2014).

5. Christoff, K., Irving, Z.C., Fox, K.C., Spreng, R.N. & Andrews-Hanna, J.R. Mind-wandering as spontaneous thought: A dynamic framework. *Nature Reviews Neuroscience* **17**, 718–731 (2016).

6. McVay, J.C. & Kane, M.J. Does mind wandering reflect executive function or executive failure? Comment on Smallwood and Schooler (2006) and Watkins (2008). *Psychological Bulletin* **136**, 188–197 (2010).

7. Diamond, A. Executive functions. *Annual Review of Psychology* **64**, 135–168 (2013).

8. Miyake, A. & Friedman, N.P. The nature and organization of individual differences in executive functions: Four general conclusions. *Current Directions in Psychological Science* **21**, 8–14 (2012).

9. Chang, Y.K., Labban, J.D., Gapin, J.I. & Etnier, J.L. The effects of acute exercise on cognitive performance: A meta-analysis. *Brain Research* **1453**, 87–101 (2012).

10. Fenesi, B., Lucibello, K., Kim, J.A. & Heisz, J.J. Sweat so you don't forget: Exercise breaks during a university lecture increase on-task attention and learning. *Journal of Applied Research in Memory and Cognition* **7**, 261–269 (2018).

11. Giles, G.E., *et al.* Acute exercise increases oxygenated and deoxygenated hemoglobin in the prefrontal cortex. *Neuroreport* **25**, 1320–1325 (2014).

12. Basso, J.C. & Suzuki, W.A. The effects of acute exercise on mood, cognition, neurophysiology, and neurochemical pathways: A review. *Brain Plasticity* **2**, 127–152 (2017).

13. Bedard, C., St John, L., Bremer, E., Graham, J.D. & Cairney, J. A systematic review and meta-analysis on the effects of physically active classrooms on educational and enjoyment outcomes in school age children. *PLOS ONE* **14**, e0218633 (2019).

14. Donnelly, J.E., *et al.* Physical activity, fitness, cognitive function, and academic achievement in children: A systematic review. *Medicine and Science in Sports and Exercise* **48**, 1197 (2016).

15. Bull, F.C., *et al.* World Health Organization 2020 guidelines on physical activity and sedentary behaviour. *British Journal of Sports Medicine* **54**, 1451–1462 (2020).

16. Ogrodnik, M., Halladay, J., Fenesi, B., Heisz, J. & Georgiades, K. Examining associations between physical activity and academic performance in a large sample of Ontario students: The role of inattention and hyperactivity. *Journal of Physical Activity and Health* **17**, 1231–1239 (2020).

17. Ng, Q.X., Ho, C.Y.X., Chan, H.W., Yong, B.Z.J. & Yeo, W.S. Managing childhood and adolescent attention-deficit/hyperactivity disorder (ADHD) with exercise: A systematic review. *Complementary Therapies in Medicine* **34**, 123–128 (2017).

18. Weyandt, L., Swentosky, A. & Gudmundsdottir, B.G. Neuroimaging and ADHD: fMRI, PET, DTI findings, and methodological limitations. *Developmental Neuropsychology* **38**, 211–225 (2013).

19. Wigal, S.B., Emmerson, N., Gehricke, J.-G. & Galassetti, P. Exercise: Applications to childhood ADHD. *Journal of Attention Disorders* **17**, 279–290 (2013).

20. Yu, C.L., *et al.* The effects of acute aerobic exercise on inhibitory control and resting state heart rate variability in children with ADHD. *Scientific Reports* **10**, 1–15 (2020).

21. Pontifex, M.B., Saliba, B.J., Raine, L.B., Picchietti, D.L. & Hillman, C.H. Exercise improves behavioral, neurocognitive, and scholastic performance in children with attention-deficit/hyperactivity disorder. *The Journal of Pediatrics* **162**, 543–551 (2013).

22. Erickson, K.I., *et al.* Physical activity, cognition, and brain outcomes: A review of the 2018 physical activity guidelines. *Medicine & Science in Sports & Exercise* **51**, 1242–1251 (2019).

23. Ludyga, S., Gerber, M., Brand, S., Holsboer-Trachsler, E. & Pühse, U. Acute effects of moderate aerobic exercise on specific aspects of executive function in different age and fitness groups: A meta-analysis. *Psychophysiology* **53**, 1611–1626 (2016).

24. Verburgh, L., Königs, M., Scherder, E.J. & Oosterlaan, J. Physical exercise and executive functions in preadolescent children, adolescents and young adults: A meta-analysis. *British Journal of Sports Medicine* **48**, 973–979 (2014).

25. Hill, E.L. Executive dysfunction in autism. *Trends in Cognitive Sciences* **8**, 26–32 (2004).

26. Bremer, E., Graham, J.D., Heisz, J.J. & Cairney, J. Effect of acute exercise on prefrontal oxygenation and inhibitory control among male children with autism spectrum disorder: An exploratory study. *Frontiers in Behavioral Neuroscience* **14**, 84 (2020).

27. Pan, C.Y., *et al.* The impacts of physical activity intervention on physical and cognitive outcomes in children with autism spectrum disorder. *Autism* **21**, 190–202 (2017).

28. Tse, C.Y.A., *et al.* Examining the impact of physical activity on sleep quality

and executive functions in children with autism spectrum disorder: A randomized controlled trial. *Autism* **23**, 1699–1710 (2019).

29. Kudrowitz, B. & Dippo, C. Getting to the novel ideas: Exploring the alternative uses test of divergent thinking. *ASME 2013 International Design Engineering Technical Conferences and Computers and Information in Engineering Conference* (American Society of Mechanical Engineers Digital Collection, 2013).

30. Feist, G.J. A meta-analysis of personality in scientific and artistic creativity. *Personality and Social Psychology Review* **2**, 290–309 (1998).

31. Richard, V., Abdulla, A.M. & Runco, M.A. Influence of skill level, experience, hours of training, and other sport participation on the creativity of elite athletes. *Journal of Genius and Eminence* **2**, 65–76 (2017).

32. Oppezzo, M. & Schwartz, D.L. Give your ideas some legs: The positive effect of walking on creative thinking. *Journal of Experimental Psychology: Learning, Memory, and Cognition* **40**, 1142 (2014).

33. Bollimbala, A., James, P. & Ganguli, S. The effect of Hatha yoga intervention on students' creative ability. *Acta Psychologica* **209**, 103121 (2020).

34. Blanchette, D.M., Ramocki, S.P., O'del, J.N. & Casey, M.S. Aerobic exercise and creative potential: Immediate and residual effects. *Creativity Research Journal* **17**, 257–264 (2005).

35. Richard, V., Abdulla, A.M. & Runco, M.A. Influence of skill level, experience, hours of training, and other sport participation on the creativity of elite athletes. *Journal of Genius and Eminence* **2**, 65–76 (2017).

36. Simons, D.J. & Chabris, C.F. Gorillas in our midst: Sustained inattentional blindness for dynamic events. *Perception* **28**, 1059–1074 (1999).

37. Memmert, D. & Furley, P. "I spy with my little eye!": Breadth of attention, inattentional blindness, and tactical decision making in team sports. *Journal of Sport and Exercise Psychology* **29**, 365–381 (2007).

38. Bowers, M.T., Green, B.C., Hemme, F. & Chalip, L. Assessing the relationship between youth sport participation settings and creativity in adulthood. *Creativity Research Journal* **26**, 314–327 (2014).

39. Dietrich, A. Neurocognitive mechanisms underlying the experience of flow. *Consciousness and Cognition* **13**, 746–761 (2004).

40. Beaty, R.E., Benedek, M., Kaufman, S.B. & Silvia, P.J. Default and executive network coupling supports creative idea production. *Scientific Reports* **5**, 1–14 (2015).

41. Arnsten, A.F. Catecholamine modulation of prefrontal cortical cognitive function. *Trends in Cognitive Sciences* **2**, 436–447 (1998).

42. Dang, L.C., O'Neil, J.P. & Jagust, W.J. Dopamine supports coupling of attention-related networks. *Journal of Neuroscience* **32**, 9582–9587 (2012).

43. Beaty, R.E., Benedek, M., Silvia, P.J. & Schacter, D.L. Creative cognition and brain network dynamics. *Trends in Cognitive Sciences* **20**, 87–95 (2016).

44. Duckworth, A.L., Peterson, C., Matthews, M.D. & Kelly, D.R. Grit: Persever-

ance and passion for long-term goals. *Journal of Personality and Social Psychology* **92**, 1087 (2007).

45. Young, B.W. & Salmela, J.H. Examination of practice activities related to the acquisition of elite performance in Canadian middle distance running. *International Journal of Sport Psychology* **41**, 73 (2010).

46. Ericsson, K.A. Towards a science of the acquisition of expert performance in sports: Clarifying the differences between deliberate practice and other types of practice. *Journal of Sports Sciences* **38**, 159–176 (2020).

47. Will Crescioni, A., *et al.* High trait self-control predicts positive health behaviors and success in weight loss. *Journal of Health Psychology* **16**, 750–759 (2011).

48. Liu-Ambrose, T., *et al.* Resistance training and executive functions: A 12-month randomized controlled trial. *Archives of Internal Medicine* **170**, 170–178 (2010).

49. Best, J.R., Nagamatsu, L.S. & Liu-Ambrose, T. Improvements to executive function during exercise training predict maintenance of physical activity over the following year. *Frontiers in Human Neuroscience* **8**, 353 (2014).

50. Antoniewicz, F. & Brand, R. Dropping out or keeping up? Early-dropouts, late-dropouts, and maintainers differ in their automatic evaluations of exercise already before a 14-week exercise course. *Frontiers in Psychology* **7**, 838 (2016).

51. Fishbach, A. & Choi, J. When thinking about goals undermines goal pursuit. *Organizational Behavior and Human Decision Processes* **118**, 99–107 (2012).

52. Wilson, K. & Brookfield, D. Effect of goal setting on motivation and adherence in a six-week exercise program. *International Journal of Sport and Exercise Psychology* **7**, 89–100 (2009).

53. Di Domenico, S.I. and Ryan, R.M. The emerging neuroscience of intrinsic motivation: A new frontier in self-determination research. *Frontiers in Human Neuroscience* **11**, 145 (2017).

54. Marashi, M.Y., *et al.* A mental health paradox: Mental health was both a motivator and barrier to physical activity during the COVID-19 pandemic. *PLOS ONE* **16(4)**, e0239244 (2021).

INDEX

Dopamine receptors, 70–75
Dorsal anterior cingulate cortex
  (dACC), 32, 35–36
Dreams, 133, 134
Driving while drowsy, 121–22
Drug(s). *See also* Addiction
  cravings for, 71, 79–80
  cues, 79
  effect on brain's reward system,
    70–71
  tolerance, 70

E
Electronic devices, 125
Elite athletes, 128
Elixir for Life workout, 116
Emotional core of pain matrix, 32
Endocannabinoids, 74–75
Endorphin Elevator, 86
Endorphins, 72–76
Endurance sports, 102
Energizers (exercise breaks), 143–44
Energy balance, in brain, 2–3
Energy balance programs, 82
Energy balance trick, 17
Episodic memory, 107, 108
Evening chronotypes, 126, 127
Executive control network, 142
Executive functions
  for achieving goals, 154–55
  improving, with exercise, 146–47,
    155–56
  three forms of, 142–43
Exercise. *See also* Exercises; Exercise
    therapy
  aerobic, 60
  alarm clock, personalizing, 127
  anti-inflammatory effects of,
    57–58
  avoiding, reasons for, 2–8
  becoming addicted to, 69
  before bedtime, 127–28
  brain's resistance to, 3–6
  brain's stress response to, 6–8

"breaks," in school settings,
    143–44
  cardiovascular, 152
  changing mindset about, 32–34
  dopamine released during, 69,
    72–75
  effect on neurogenesis, 106
  effect on PNS and SNS, 59–60
  effect on sleep quality, 123–24
  finding the right intensity, 8–11
  with friends, 110
  group-based, 75–76
  increasing enjoyment for, 11–13
  intense, recovering from, 16
  lack of harm from, 37
  mental health mode of, 63–64
  scheduling time for, 5–6
  and sleep deprivation, 122
  slow and steady approach to, 13,
    16–17
  workout times, matching chrono-
    type with, 125–27
  World Health Organization recom-
    mendations on, 144–45
Exercise pill, 109
Exercises
  Arm Circles (backward), 167
  Arm Circles (forward), 167
  Arm Swings (across the body), 168
  Arm Swings (up and down), 168
  Bicycles, 169
  Bird Dogs, 169
  Butt Kicks, 170
  Cat Cow, 171
  Crossovers, 172
  Dead Bugs, 173
  Deadlifts, 174
  Front Plank, 175
  Front Plank (modified), 175
  Heel Walk, 176
  High Knees, 176
  Hip Openers, 177
  Hip Twists, 177
  Jumping Jacks, 178